SEXUALLY TRANSMITTED DISEASES

Dr David Plummer
Professor Gabor Kovacs
Ann Westmore

HILL OF CONTENT
Melbourne

First published in Australia 1995
by Hill of Content Publishing
86 Bourke Street
MELBOURNE 3000

Cover design: The Letterbox
Typeset by: Midland Typesetters, Maryborough, Victoria
Printed by: Australian Print Group, Maryborough, Victoria

National Library Cataloguing-in-publication

Plummer, David, 1957-
   Sexually transmitted diseases

   Includes index.
   ISBN 0 85572 249 5.

1. Sexually transmitted diseases. I. Kovacs, Gabor, 1947-
II. Westmore, Ann, 1953-   . III. Title.

616.951

CONTENTS

Introduction   iv

1   A Journey Around the Genital Region   1

2   How Infectious Organisms Work: Key Principles   9

3   Sex in the Real World   23

4   Springing Leaks—Genital Discharges   33

5   Lumps, Bumps, Warts and All   49

6   Blisters, Ulcers, Abrasions, Raw Areas and Scabs   57

7   Red & Itchy Areas   69

8   Sexually Transmitted Infections that Travel in the   78
    Bloodstream

9   STD's and Sexual Health   104

    Suggested Further Reading   118

    Index   119

INTRODUCTION

This book is intended for individuals and health professionals who need to know more about sexually transmitted diseases (STDs). While readers will find a level of detail that is not generally available in books on this subject, we have attempted to provide this information in a clear and accessible way using plain english. We do not accept the common practice of providing two versions of every medical problem: one for the doctor and a patronisingly simplified version for patients that tends to distort or omit relevant information.

The opening chapters provide background information on anatomy, physiology and microbiology for people with little knowledge of the health sciences or who want a refresher, while the core of the book is devoted to STDs themselves. These core chapters are written from the viewpoint of how problems reveal themselves to patients and to their clinicians.

Using as starting points the symptoms that individuals complain of, and the signs that health workers uncover on examination and testing, the book leads the reader to the likely diagnosis and to the actions likely to prove most helpful.

This 'syndromic' approach—rather than the classic 'scientific' approach that begins with organisms and biology—is intended to enhance the readability and usefulness of the book.

For lay readers as well as those well-grounded in the health sciences, we have set out the cornerstones of STD practice, devoting particular attention to areas where traps and errors commonly occur.

In addition, experiences of actual patients are included to help readers relate the information provided to real life. These stories are not intended to answer questions, but to raise them by documenting people's experiences. Of course, we have altered names to protect the privacy of the individuals concerned.

David Plummer, Gab Kovacs, Ann Westmore.

Chapter One

A JOURNEY AROUND THE GENITAL REGION

'I wish I'd known more about my body and the havoc that
sexually transmitted diseases can cause before I got involved.
I'm convinced I'd be happier and healthier if I'd been
acquainted with the facts earlier.'

Hurt, shocked, scared, angry, regretful.

These are the sorts of words people use to sum up how they feel when told they have a sexually transmitted disease (STD).

It is not just the physical symptoms and their possible consequence that cause stress and distress.

STDs strike deep into the individual psyche and can have a permanently disabling effect if emotional as well as physical aspects are not addressed.

This book tackles the mesh of issues associated with STDs. It recognises that while prevention is the ideal, many people are at risk of STD infection at some stage if they are at all sexually active.

Words alone cannot hope to rid the body of the impact of disease. But accurate, understandable information is an essential first step towards protection from STDs. In addition, if disease transmission is suspected, sound information helps us decide if our concerns are justified, who to turn to for advice or help, and the sorts of testing and treatments available.

Men and women are not reproductive machines or sensory organs on stilts. Their behaviour is the result of complex needs, emotions, attitudes and beliefs. Thus, while this chapter explores the relationship between the human body and STDs, it should be seen as background information for the personal dramas that can take place in situations of personal intimacy.

In the descriptions that follow it is important to realise that no

1

two people have exactly the same genital geography (unless, perhaps, they are identical twins). The range of 'normal' in genital size, shape, contour and texture is enormous and the chance that any structure is abnormal is small. If, despite this reassurance, you are concerned about some aspect of your body, it is advisable to have it checked by an experienced medical practitioner.

A woman's genital geography

Women's external and internal sexual organs complement each other well.

The external organs, collectively known as the vulva, seem designed for 'show and feel' purposes. In contrast, the internal organs are the engine-room that drive the monthly menstrual cycle and provide the setting for the development of the unborn baby.

The word vulva has its origins in the Latin word for 'wrapper'. Its most immediately obvious part is the labia majora (large or outer lips), the two soft folds of skin covered with pubic hair.

On parting the legs, two finer hairless lips, the labia minora, are visible on the inner surface of the labia majora.

The clitoris, a small pink nob of firmer tissue with a profound ability to produce pleasant sensations, can also be seen. A highly touch-sensitive tissue, the clitoris increases in size and deepens in colour (due to an inflow of blood) with sexual arousal.

Just below the clitoris and between the labia minora is a small opening (the urethra) for the passage of urine. Below this again is the larger entrance of the vagina (derived from the Latin for 'sheath').

Beyond the vulva and between the buttocks is the opening of the anus.

On the inside

The vagina is well constructed to cope with the rigours of childbirth and lovemaking. Layer upon layer of flat (squamous) cells ensure it can flex and stretch as required. Bands of muscular tissue surrounding these lining cells enable the vagina to mould itself around fingers, a tampon, a penis or a baby during birth.

The hymen, or what remains of it, lies just inside the entrance to the vagina. It is a thin curtain of tissue that partially blocks the vagina or lies flattened against its wall. This flattening may occur in various ways including tampon usage or intercourse.

The vagina is naturally moist due to the presence of numerous glands around and within it. Although the glands are not visible to the naked eye, they are capable of ample lubrication. They produce increased amounts of moisture at times of sexual excitement, even when distant parts of the body are touched (such as the nipples). The main moisturising glands are called Bartholin's glands and the para-urethral glands. As well as providing lubrication, their secretions help keep the vagina clean and maintain a level of acidity that minimises the chances of infection.

The innermost portion of the vagina merges with the cervix (or neck of the uterus/womb). The cervix is composed of fibrous tissue and has two main parts as follows:

* the outer cervix (ectocervix), which is covered with a layer of the same type of flat cells that line the vagina
* the inner cervix (endocervix), which forms a canal and is lined with a single layer of tall cells interspersed with many glands. The endocervix seems particularly prone to infection by organisms that may be sexually transmitted, perhaps because of its glandular architecture.

The dividing line between the ectocervix and the endocervix is known as the transformation zone. It is an area that tends to be unstable, the most likely site of cervical cancer. For this reason, a sample of cells for a Pap smear must include some cells from this zone. (Similarly, the anus has two distinct cell types, at the junction of which cancers of the rectum predominantly occur.) All women who are sexually active are advised to have a Pap smear (see Chapter 9) at least every two years up to age 70.

The cervix forms the lower part of the uterus (also known as the womb), which resembles a small hollow pear, pointed downwards. A thick layer of muscle (the myometrium) allows the uterus to act as a strong yet flexible chamber that is 'home' to the developing baby should pregnancy occur.

The inside lining of the uterus (the endometrium) is a marvel of nature. Its quick-growing cells build up over a couple of weeks and then disintegrate unless they are needed to provide nourishment and support to a pregnancy. If this is not required, the endometrial tissue and blood (the menstrual flow or menstruation) pass from the body several days usually about once a month.

Judith considered herself to be a lucky woman. She met her first serious boyfriend when she was 17 and married him four years later. She and her husband had an exuberant sexual relationship and two beautiful children.

At the age of 33 she became concerned at the amount of vaginal discharge she sometimes produced during her menstrual cycle. The discharge seemed to have increased since the birth of her second child and she sought advice from her doctor on several occasions. Each time he took samples for testing, but the result was always the same—'no abnormal organisms present.'

Eventually Judith's doctor sent her to a gynaecologist who examined her and explained that her cervix was very active and made lots of mucous. The doctor said this was a normal secretion of the cervix and was important for lubricating the vagina and keeping it free from infection. This reassurance put Judith's worries to rest and she later realised how fortunate she was. Several girlfriends with whom she discussed the matter wished they had her problem. They said they sometimes experienced a dry vagina which made sex far from comfortable.

This build up/break down sequence results in the typical menstrual cycle pattern and the entire process is controlled by hormones (chemical messenger substances) released from organs including the ovaries and the brain. The ovaries, a pair of organs about the size and shape of two almonds, contain and nurture eggs (also known as ova), the female sex cells. Baby girls are born with several hundred thousand immature eggs in their ovaries. Between puberty (when periods start) and the menopause (when they stop), several hundred of these eggs mature and burst from the ovary, usually one at a time and at approximately monthly intervals.

After each menstrual period, a crop of eggs starts to develop, with one egg usually taking the lead. When it is fully mature, it bursts from the ovary in the process known as ovulation. For a short time it hovers in the gap between an ovary and its nearby Fallopian tube which provides a potential passageway to the uterus. The mature egg is usually swept into the end of the Fallopian tube nearest the ovary by finger-like projections (called fimbriae) soon after ovulation. The delicate nature of the fimbriae makes them susceptible to damage by sexually transmitted, or other, infectious organisms.

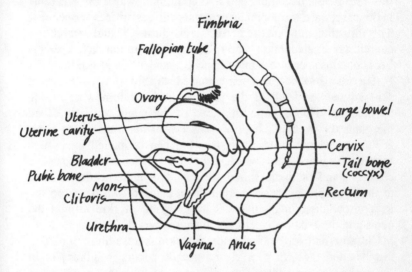

Anatomy of female genital organs

Hormones help make it happen

There are two common ways in which messages are sent from one body part to another. The first is along nerve pathways, for example, from the brain to the thigh and back again. The second message system involves chemical messenger substances called hormones which are produced in many parts of the body and which can have a powerful impact a long way from their source after transportation by the blood or lymph drainage system. Sex hormones are one important group of such substances and they exert a profound effect on the genital organs, for example, stimulating the production of various secretions. The presence of such secretions may, in turn, influence the spread of STDs.

The hormones, oestrogen and progesterone, are particularly important in this regard and we will look at them more closely in later chapters.

Mapping a man's sexual parts

The most obvious part of a man's reproductive equipment is the penis, a multi-purpose organ that is highly sensitive to touch. Normally the penis is soft and limp but, with sexual arousal, it fills with blood, becoming stiff and pointing upwards (an erection). In this erect state, the penis can penetrate various orifices or openings. The thrusting movements of the penis during sexual intercourse can climax in ejaculation and release of a secretion called semen. This contains sperm (the male sex cells), and a mix of fluids.

If a man has not been circumcised, the foreskin (a sleeve of skin around the head of the penis) rolls back somewhat during an erection. This exposes the head of the penis which is called the glans (or fireman's helmet). The rim of the head of the penis is known as the corona. The foreskin can be pulled back fully to reveal the whole glans which is covered with delicate and sensitive cells. A band of tissue called the frenulum underneath the head of the penis prevents the foreskin from being drawn back too far. In a circumcised man, there is no covering of skin around the penis and these delicate cells are always exposed.

Circumcision or removal of the foreskin is a tradition in certain families and races of people, and usually occurs in infancy or in the early teenage years. The debate about whether circumcision has any advantages in terms of better hygiene is on-going with some studies suggesting there may be an increased risk of some STDs in particular groups of uncircumcised men. The weight of medical opinion supports the view that the regular drawing back of the foreskin and washing and drying of the glans, avoids problems.

The other role of the penis is to pass urine. Whereas in women, urine passes from the body through its own separate passage, in men the penis serves as a pathway for urine as well as sperm. The tube connecting the bladder to the tip or eye of the penis (the urethral meatus) is called the urethra. On its way from the bladder to the tip of the penis, the urethra passes through the prostate gland, a chestnut-shaped organ at the base of the bladder. When a man is sexually excited, the sperm and other secretions, collectively called the semen, enter the urethra ready for ejaculation. The prostate can be a source of pleasure for some people and is responsible for much of the fluid in semen. Thus men who have had prostate surgery can expect to produce a reduced volume of semen. Some

STDs result in an unpleasant discharge from the urethra and they may do sufficient damage to it to cause narrowing and difficulty in passing urine.

Apart from the penis, the other male sexual organs that are permanently outside his body are the testicles. These lie in a pouch called the scrotum between the legs. The testicles, two oval structures which ache when squeezed, are the factories for sperm production. The testicles and penis are linked by an array or tubes that tend to be vulnerable to infection by STDs, leading to obstruction and the possibility of sterility. Within the testicles themselves is a convoluted system of small tubes. These merge into the epididymis (the main storage site of sperm) and then into two larger tubes known as the vas deferens. Attached to each vas just before it enters the prostate gland are two other glands called seminal vesicles. They add nourishing secretions to the sperm as it waits to be ejaculated, thereby increasing the volume of the semen.

At the base of the bladder, an intricate valve system acts like a three-way tap to the penis. When ejaculation is about to occur, the tap closes off the bladder so that urine is not released and the semen can pass along the penis.

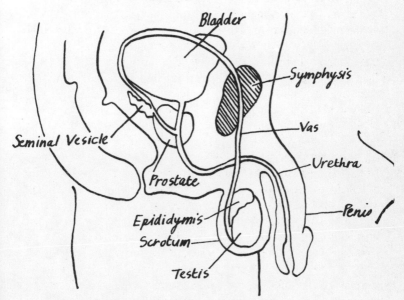

Anatomy of male genital organs

Testosterone and the male reproductive system

As well as producing sperm, the testicles have another important function. They manufacture the sex hormone, testosterone, which gradually decreases in amount from around the age of puberty to old age. Testosterone is essential for the development of male characteristics like hair growth, a deep voice and typical male body shape. It also helps maintain normal function of the sexual organs and influences libido (interest in sex). Lack of testosterone results in difficulty with erection, decreased body hair and a higher pitch of the voice.

It is quite common for the sperm-producing ability of the testicles to be damaged without affecting testosterone production or other aspects of sexual behaviour. Thus men who are sterile (incapable of fathering a child), for example because of STD-induced damage to the testicles, may have an active interest in sex and an ongoing ability to achieve erections.

Chapter Two

HOW INFECTIOUS ORGANISMS WORK: KEY PRINCIPLES

Misunderstandings about sexually transmitted diseases (STDs) frequently stem from ignorance or confusion about the ways that infectious organisms work and their interactions with humans to cause disease.

As the term implies, STDs are transmitted by sexual contact from a person with an existing infection to a person who is not yet infected. Sexual contact is not confined to penetration of the vagina by the penis. It can also include mouth-to-mouth kissing, contact between the mouth and vagina or the mouth and the penis, and anal intercourse.

STDs are notoriously difficult to eradicate from the community because they may not produce easily recognisable symptoms, especially in the early stages of infection. This is why STDs are sometimes described as 'silent'. Carriers of an infection may not realise, initially or ever, that they are infected and that they pose a health risk to others. The absence of adequate diagnosis, treatment and/or education may also contribute to the persistence of infection for life, further adding to the pool of STDs in the community.

Infections: How they work

Infections are caused by living organisms (loosely termed germs) so small that, at best, they can be seen only under a microscope. Various characteristics of organisms have lead scientists to divide them into four basic groups—viruses, bacteria, fungi and parasites.

Like all living things including people, the viruses, bacteria, fungi and parasites have their own set of in-built instructions containing all the information needed for survival. This 'master control' is known as the genetic code and its main components are the nucleic acids.

A handful of key nucleic acids form an elaborate code by linking together in inumerable different combinations. A group of three nucleic acids is called a triplet or codon and forms the basis of the code. The chains formed by linking these codons together are known as DNA and RNA (DeoxyriboNucleic Acid and RiboNucleic Acid). The coded DNA chain resembles a compact spiral and is known as the 'double helix'.

The sole function of DNA is to act as a memory that provides a blueprint to construct the building blocks of life. These building blocks are proteins and they have two main functions.

One is to form a scaffolding that gives the living thing its characteristic shape. Proteins with this role are known as structural proteins. Our bones, hair and skin gain their shape from this type of protein.

The second function of proteins is to enable cells to operate efficiently. Proteins that carry out this function are known as enzymes and they regulate the day to day activities of living things. The contraction of muscles, digestion and the activities of the brain are examples of functions that depend on enzymes.

The genetic code, the structural proteins and the enzymes float in a salty fluid surrounded by a membrane—a bit like a plastic bag full of salt water. This is an outline of a cell. Animals and humans are made of billions of cells, whereas bacteria, fungi and most of the parasites that cause STDs consist of only one cell.

Viruses form a special category. Rather than existing as an entire cell, they are pure nucleic acid packaged inside a protein coat.

Viruses, bacteria, fungi and parasites

Viruses are considered to be the simplest of the infectious agents but this does not mean they are easy to control. They are inactive until they attach to a cell and enter it. They then hijack the cell by closing down the cell's normal genetic code and directing activities according to their own genetic code. The cell becomes a factory for making copies of the virus and, in many cases, once this function is complete the cell dies. Alternately, the virus may enter the cell and lie dormant for prolonged periods before becoming active and causing a disease.

The net result of viral infection is the production of millions of new virus particles. These are released either by budding from the surface of the cell or by causing the cell to burst. Viruses that bud from the surface, take with them into the world a coating or envelope made from the cell membrane. Proteins belonging to the virus are added to the envelope forming a partnership that is essential for further viral transmission. Such viruses can be rendered harmless by damaging the envelope. However standard antibiotic treatments are ineffective against them.

Examples of STDs caused by viruses include warts, herpes, glandular fever, hepatitis B, hepatitis C and AIDS. The virus that causes AIDS is known as HIV (Human Immunodeficiency Virus). Both the herpes virus and HIV are enveloped which makes them potentially more vulnerable to human control than some other viruses.

Bacteria are more sophisticated than viruses but are arguably less elegant. Bacteria are complete cells and can usually function independently of a living host. While this has some advantages for them it also means they can be grown successfully in the laboratory and can be damaged or destroyed by antibiotics.

In the past, some bacteria were mistaken for viruses because, while carrying out some functions independently, these bacteria relied on living cells for their survival. One such sexually transmitted organism is chlamydia which depends on cells to provide it with energy.

Other bacteria such as gonorrhoea and syphilis also have special requirements for growth which helps explain why laboratory testing and diagnosis may be difficult. Gonorrhoea requires a higher than normal carbon dioxide level and added vitamins if it is to grow successfully on agar plates. (Agar is an inert, jelly-like substance which provides a moist, solid base suitable for the growth of many organisms in the laboratory.) Syphilis is not yet grown successfully in the laboratory as its special growth requirements have yet to be identified.

Fungi are higher forms of life than bacteria and can be divided into two groups. The first, **yeasts**, form moist, creamy colonies when grown in the laboratory at body temperature. Examples of yeasts include candida and cryptococcus.

Although candida can cause vaginal and penile infections (thrush), the candida yeast is normally resident in the intestine and is not usually transmitted by sex. Candida and cryptococcus are common in people with AIDS. They respond to antifungal drugs but not to antibiotics. Both can be grown successfully on agar plates.

The second group of fungi are known as **moulds**. When grown in the laboratory they form long filaments that mesh together like a pad of cotton-wool. The most common moulds seen in the STD clinic are those that cause tinea, a fungal infection of skin, hair or nails. Such skin-loving moulds are known as dermatophytes.

Some **parasites** can also cause STDs. Included in this group are small, single cell parasites known as protozoa and larger organisms made up of many cells including pin worm, lice (a six legged insect) and scabies (an eight legged mite). Protozoal infections include trichomonas which can invade the vagina. Examples of parasites that occur in association with AIDS include pneumocystis, toxoplasma and cryptosporidium.

The source and spread of infections

Infections do not simply appear from nowhere. They can only occur if there is contact with a disease-causing organism. In the case of STDs, this usually means contact with an infection that is found in the genital area and is passed from person to person by sexual contact.

Why are STDs transmitted during sex while other infections are passed by coughing or by ingesting food or water? The explanation lies in the makeup of the different organisms and especially the nature of the proteins on their outer surfaces.

The surfaces of the organisms that cause STDs are covered with proteins that match proteins on the surface of genital cells. On coming into contact, these fit like a lock and key, and the organism attaches itself to the genital cell.

Some infections such as chlamydia and gonorrhoea specifically target the lining cells of the cervix and urethra. Their transmission requires direct contact between an infected cell on for example, the eye of the penis, with cells of the cervix or urethra. Thus intimate sexual contact is always involved in their spread.

The opportunities for some other infections, such as wart virus infections, to enter the body are more numerous as they may lock on to surface proteins on skin or moist mucus membranes.

Some STDs infect the blood and/or other tissues some distance from the genitals and then pass into genital fluids. From there they can be transmitted by latching on to another individual's mucus membranes. Examples of infections of this type include hepatitis B, hepatitis C, HIV and syphilis. Different fluids from the same person may behave in different ways as far as carriage of the STD organism goes. For example, if some saliva from an individual infected with HIV enters the healthy mouth of another person this does not seem to result in spread of the infection unless a cut, ulcer or lesion is present in that person's mouth. Whereas if semen or vaginal fluids from someone with HIV enters the mouth of the uninfected person, there appears to be a low risk of transmission.

The notion that STDs are transmitted via toilet seats and the like is widespread. While casual contact with toilet seats and other inanimate objects has not been linked with STD transmission, it is reasonable not to share sex toys or anything that could be contaminated with fresh genital secretions and that could come into contact with susceptible parts of the anatomy such as the moist surfaces of the penis, vulva or vagina. Likewise, it is reasonable to observe good handwashing procedures when dealing with blood and other body fluids and, in particular, to avoid accidents with sharp objects that are contaminated with fresh blood. It is also reasonable to avoid sharing razors with someone who is infected with HIV or hepatitis.

On the other hand, it is not reasonable to avoid shaking hands with a person who has AIDS as this carries no risk of disease transmission. It is also unreasonable to blame mosquitoes for the spread of AIDS for, while they are known to spread certain diseases, there are good biological explanations for why AIDS and most other infections are not among them.

It is important to realise that not all infections involving the genitals are sexually transmitted. Some infections such as skin infections can attack the skin anywhere including the genitals. Examples of bacteria which can infect the genitals but which are not necessarily sexually transmitted include staphylococci and streptococci (staphs and streps), thrush (candida) and gardnerella. Infection may occur because of some local disturbance, for example, due to rubbing or dampness. This may allow the organism access to some cells, perhaps resulting in symptoms such as redness, itchiness or a rash.

Some people who are infected do not show signs of infection immediately or at all. People who are infected but symptom-free are called 'carriers'. For example, people with HIV may carry the virus with few if any symptoms for many years before serious illness occurs. Similarly, the serious consequences of genital wart virus infection may take many years to become apparent or may never do so despite the life-long nature of wart virus infection. Chlamydia infection is also often silent, yet during this time of silence, a woman who harbours the organisms may sustain damage to her Fallopian tubes with resultant infertility.

The silent nature of some STD infections helps explain the failure of strategies that rely totally on people with symptoms seeking treatment.

Immunity and sexually transmitted diseases

The immune system is our defence against invasion by infections and depends on white blood cells known as lymphocytes. When these cells come into contact with a foreign invader (such as an infectious organism), they react and develop 'memory' cells that can recognise the invader in the future and thus quickly trigger an immune reaction. Only small fragments of the invaders are needed to trigger the immune response. These fragments are called 'antigens'.

The two main types of lymphocyte responsible for defending the body against invaders are known as T cells and B cells. The presence of a foreign antigen causes T cells to activate and coordinate the immune response. This in turn results in activation of B cells and production by them of substances known as antibodies.

Antibodies are proteins capable of changing their structure, thus enabling them to match and react with parts of the original invader. They can attach to the invader and inactivate it or trigger a sequence of events that destroys it.

T cells control immunity by releasing a number of messengers that stimulate various cells to attack the invader. They can be divided into two key types known as T4 (or CD4) and T8 (or CD8) cells. T 4 cells are also known as 'helper' cells for their ability to coordinate and stimulate an adequate immune response. T8 cells are known as 'suppressor' cells because they are capable of damping down the immune response. Helper and suppressor T cells delicately balance the task of producing an immune response that is neither too vigorous nor too weak.

A key to understanding sexually transmitted infections is that the body's ability to defend itself against them is often imperfect. For example, HIV silently destroys the helper T cells and, in this situation of immune system impairment, other infections take the opportunity to enter the body. This ultimately results in the symptoms of AIDS. Syphilis, on the other hand, stimulates an immune response which, although not usually enough to eradicate the infection, can cause quite serious damage. Indeed, most of the long-term problems associated with syphilis are thought to be due to the immune response itself rather than the syphilis!

In the case of hepatitis B, most adults who become infected have a bout of hepatitis and are then able to clear the virus. However, about 5% of infected individuals are unable to overcome the infection and these people often 'carry' the virus for the rest of their lives, some eventually developing serious liver damage. Chlamydia escapes the immune system by concealing itself inside the cells of the person it infects. Gonnorrhoea can also evade the immune response by hiding its antigens. As with a number of infections, individuals who come into contact with gonorrhoea can become infected repeatedly—each time they come into contact with the responsible organism.

Ineffective immune responses would not matter so much if vaccines were available to stimulate effective immunity. Unfortunately, scientists have not been able to develop vaccines against most STDs. A major exception is the development of a vaccine against hepatitis B which uses a purified component of the surface of the hepatitis B virus known as the hepatitis B surface antigen. Three doses of this vaccine over six months generates an effective immune response in about 95% of people who are vaccinated.

In the absence of vaccines against other STDs, the best protection is prevention.

Tests: principles

There are three basic types of test that are used to detect STDs; tests for whole organisms, tests for fragments of organisms (antigens) and tests for a response by the body to the infection (antibodies). A broad understanding of how these tests work provides many useful insights into the nature of infections and how the body responds to them.

Tests for whole organisms typically involve examinations of samples under a microscope and growth (culture) of any organisms found. The sample used may be obtained by collecting a small amount of abnormal fluid (discharge) from the eye of the penis or from the vagina. If the discharge is examined while moist and fresh, the test is called a 'wet preparation'. If the smear is dried and then stained, the test is known as a gram stain. Wet preparations are useful for checking urine and for looking for trichomonas in vaginal discharges. Gram stains are particularly useful for diagnosing thrush, gonorrhoea and gardnerella. These tests typically take around 10 minutes. Thus it is often possible to make an accurate diagnosis and to start effective treatment almost immediately.

Some infectious organisms are too small to be seen under an ordinary microscope and special measures have to be taken to detect them. Syphilis is smaller than most bacteria and needs a modified microscope called a 'dark-ground' microscope. This is a standard microscope but the light is beamed in such a way that the organism responsible for syphilis is seen as a bright spiral swimming against a dark background. This technique is particularly useful in early syphilis before blood tests are reliably positive.

Viruses can only be seen with a very high powered microscope called an electron microscope. Using this sort of equipment, the virus responsible for herpes can be detected at an early stage when typical fluid-filled blisters are present. Because 'dark-ground' and electron microscopes tend to be available only in specialised clinics, it is more usual to use other methods to show evidence of syphilis and viruses.

Blood tests can be used to look for either fragments of an infection (antigens) or the body's response to infection (antibodies). Because antibodies match the foreign parts (antigens) of the invader exactly, they can be used as markers of contact with an infection, even if the body has since eliminated the infection. Like a footprint in the sand, the evidence is still there after the beachcomber has left the beach. Antibodies give an indication that there has been an immune response but they do not necessarily indicate its effectiveness. For example the AIDS antibody test indicates contact with HIV as well as permanent infection. In general, specific antibodies last for life but some infections also cause less specific antibodies that do not last for life. In the case of syphilis, the less specific test, the 'RPR test' becomes negative a year or two after successful treatment, while the specific tests remain permanently positive. The RPR is therefore useful to check that the treatment has worked. (RPR stands for Rapid Plasma Reagin test: so called, because it is a rapid blood test for the non-specific antibodies against syphilis called 'reagin'.)

The body can produce a range of antibodies against different components of the same organism and these may provide different information. For example, antibodies against the surface of the hepatitis B virus indicate that the person has resolved the infection and is protected, whereas antibodies against the core of the hepatitis B virus alone may be found while the virus is still present.

Finally, there can be different types of antibodies against the same component of the infecting organism and these may be useful too. In the case of hepatitis B, the antibody against the core of the virus comes in two main forms. One core antibody, IgM, indicates that the infection was recent. This antibody disappears during the few months after the infection and is replaced with IgG which remains positive for life. These two components can therefore provide some idea as to whether the infection was recent or not.

Tests for antigens are tests for components of the organisms that cause infections. These tests can be done on blood and some should be done on samples from other sites. For example, samples from the urethra of men or the cervix in women can be tested for chlamydia antigen. Unfortunately, as described later, these tests can be difficult to perform and must be interpreted with care.

Tests: problems

Nowadays, technology is seen as the answer to most of humanity's problems. However, it is important to realise that medical tests are far from perfect and caution must be exercised when interpreting the results. Too often, doctors blindly accept test results at face value. The following general points illustrate some of the problems.

There is always a lag period between the time a person becomes infected and the time that a test can detect the infection. This is known as the window period and varies between a few days for some tests to three months for others. The window period explains why it is usually not possible to give an 'all clear' to people who may have been exposed recently to an infectious organism. This is also the main reason why certificates giving a 'clean bill of health' should not be given to people who have been tested unless the window period is well and truly over. Another reason is that the certificates start to go out of date from the day the tests are taken and it is perfectly possible for a person to pick up an infection before the results are back from the laboratory.

Tests are only as good as the specimens that are collected from patients. This is particularly so for some STDs because the organisms are often fragile once they leave the comfortable environment of the body. Special methods of collecting specimens and of testing have therefore been developed for most STDs. As with any system, clerical and laboratory mistakes can occur and it is vitally important that testing procedures are carefully followed and that all specimens are correctly labelled. This may be regarded as a nuisance at the time, but it is essential if an accurate result is to be achieved.

There is always a chance that test results are incorrect. False positive tests mean that the test gives a positive result even though the person is not infected. False positives occur in around one in every ten positive tests for chlamydia antigen. Regrettably, false negative tests (where the test is negative even though the person is infected) also occur. Again, with chlamydia it is not uncommon for the test to miss the infection even though symptoms are apparent. Possible explanations for false negatives are that the test was taken from a spot where the infection was no longer active, the test was taken incorrectly, the chlamydia died on the way to the laboratory or the test was simply too insensitive to detect the organism.

Every test has certain levels of sensitivity and specificity. Sensitivity refers to how well the test can detect an infection. Most tests are not 100% sensitive and will miss some infections. Specificity refers to how precisely the test picks up a particular organism. Most tests are not 100% specific and will occasionally give a positive result when a person does not have an infection. The chance of a positive test being accurate is known as the positive predictive value. The chance of a negative test being accurate is called the negative predictive value. To complicate things even further these values depend on how common an infection is in a population!

Confused? The best way to understand these problems is to look at HIV tests. These are nearly 100% specific but positive results are always double checked with a 'western blot' test. HIV tests are also very sensitive but false negatives can occur and there is a 'window period' before the test starts to show positive results. By repeating the test three months after possible exposure to the virus, the window period is covered. This makes testing more sensitive.

To illustrate how the predictive value of a test depends on who is being tested let us look at two population groups. People who donate blood have a very low risk of HIV infection. Very rarely, however, the blood bank finds donated blood that tests HIV positive. It discards the blood and follows up the donor. Often, the test turns

Elisa AIDs test. detects
HIV-1 only (not HIV-2)

out to be a false positive and the donor is found not to have the infection. Therefore the 'positive predictive value' of the HIV test at the blood bank (the chance that a positive test accurately predicts that the person is positive) is low.

On the other hand, there is a much bigger chance that a positive test at an STD clinic or a clinic for people on methadone (used as a substitute for heroin) is a true positive because the people being tested have a relatively high risk of HIV infection. In this setting, the positive predictive value of the same test is high!

All medical tests have similar pitfalls but some are more accurate than others. The important message is not to jump to conclusions. It is very important to ask about the likelihood of a test result being correct and to assess the information provided. Whatever the result of a test, a good clinical assessment is vital.

STD treatments: some guidelines

Good treatment of STDs is more than just prescribing drugs. A relationship of trust between the health worker and the patient is crucial. A clear and reassuring explanation is always helpful—but is frequently inadequate or overlooked. Patients need to understand what is going on in order to make decisions and to have some control over what is happening. Feeling out of control can often intensify the trauma of STD diagnosis and treatment. People who do not want to know about STDs may have misguided notions and may continue to put themselves and others at risk. Gentle inquiry into a person's ideas and attitudes may reveal important problems that should be addressed.

The diagnosis of a sexually related infection often has implications for an individual's attitude to sex from then on. Dealing with negative feelings about sexuality may be timely. STD diagnosis also has important implications for partners and relationships, and ensuring appropriate and sensitive handling of contacts and partners is essential.

As a general principle, it is always important to ensure that partners are treated: that precautions are taken during treatment to ensure that others do not become infected or reinfected: and that courses of treatment are completed. The aim is to help the person feel better, to eradicate the infection, to prevent complications and to prevent further spread. Reinfection may occur if precautions are not followed from the time of starting treatment to the time of final checkup, if partners are not correctly treated, or if treatment is incomplete.

Treatments can be divided into specific and non-specific measures. Non-specific treatments include pain relief; counselling to reduce anxiety and to improve understanding and a sense of control; soothing creams; and so forth. Specific treatments include antibiotics and other measures to control the infection. In general antibiotics, are only active against bacteria. Bacterial infections that can be treated with antibiotics include chlamydia, gonorrhoea, syphilis, gardnerella and urinary infections. Each of these infections requires treatment with a different antibiotic.

Some medications can cause side-effects and these should be explained at the time they are prescribed. For example, metronidazole should not be taken with alcohol because unpleasant reactions such as nausea and stomach cramps can occur. Some antibiotics like doxycycline and erythromycin can cause nausea, and thus should be taken on a full stomach and washed down with water to minimise these problems.

Acyclovir and AZT are antiviral drugs that are sometimes prescribed in STD clinics for herpes and HIV respectively. Antiviral drugs act in a different way to antibiotics. Basically, they interfere with the copying process of the virus' nucleic acid code. Some antivirals have side-effects because they can also interact with the nucleic acid code of the patient. Others, like acyclovir seem to be almost completely free of side-effects because they only become active in cells that contain the virus.

Antifungal treatments are used against candida, which causes thrush, the dermatophytes that cause tinea and cryptococcus which causes infections of the blood, bones, brain and lungs in AIDS. Because thrush and tinea develop on moist surfaces and skin, the medication is usually added to a cream which is rubbed into the infected area. Antifungal drugs for vaginal thrush come in both cream and pessary forms. Pessaries are vaginal tablets and have the same effect as the cream but some people find them easier to use. The pessary is made of a wax such as paraffin which 'melts' in the vagina, releasing the therapy. Antifungal drugs are also produced in tablet form, but most are useless against vaginal thrush because they are not absorbed into the blood and do not reach the vagina.

Although trichomonas is a parasite, it responds to an antibiotic called metronidazole which also works against some bacteria. It is not surprising to find that scabies and lice (mites and insects respectively) respond to insecticides. Most domestic insecticides are too irritating or toxic to use directly on people, but the standard treatments are basically safe insecticides in a moisturising cream, rubbed into the infected area.

Prevention

Prevention is always superior to relying on diagnosis and treatment. People may not suspect they have infections, may be too afraid to seek help, tests may miss the diagnosis and some infections are resistant to treatment or are untreatable.

Safe sex is not just for AIDS prevention. Other common STDs also have potentially serious consequences but people are less aware of them. Prolonged carriage of hepatitis B or C viruses can result in liver damage and cirrhosis; wart virus has been linked to cancer of the cervix; genital herpes has been associated with severe infections in the newborn and untreated syphilis can cause brain and heart damage. All of these complications can be fatal but STDs can have other serious but non-fatal complications such as infertility, ruined relationships, misery, depression and sexual hangups.

The aim of prevention is to place an effective barrier between individuals and the infection. In effect this is a form of quarantine, but instead of quarantining the person, it is often possible to quarantine the infection. A barrier can be created by deciding not to have sex or by having sexual contact that does not include intercourse, having only one safe partner or using condoms. All of these methods reduce the risk of aquiring a range of infections, and the method(s) used will depend on the individuals involved and their circumstances. The word 'individual' is used deliberately because in the case of voluntary activities, it only takes one partner to decide to be safe.

All of these preventive methods also have shortcomings. Not having sex (celibacy or abstinence) seems to be the choice of relatively few people. Reducing the number of partners probably decreases the chances of becoming infected, but it must be remembered that it only takes one unsafe contact to pass on an infection. Likewise, having only one safe partner (monogamy) is safe in theory but is limited by the partners that you and your partner have had previously and by your continuing 'faithfulness' to each other. Indeed, in our community, the failure of monogamy may well be higher than the failure of condoms! Most importantly, because there is no 'typical' patient and because most STDs can be silent, there is no easy way to detect who has an STD. Making assumptions about people is unreliable and is a form of risk-taking.

It seems sensible to always add condoms for safety. Condoms used properly seem to provide good protection against HIV, chlamydia and gonorrhoea. Because condoms are impenetrable to viruses, they should also reduce the chances of contracting herpes provided an area of infection can be sufficiently covered. On the other hand, condoms are less effective against hepatitis B because the infective agent can occasionally be passed in saliva.

Chapter Three

SEX IN THE REAL WORLD

When the English First Fleet sailed into Botany Bay, south of present day Sydney, in 1788 so did some troublesome STDs.

The entries of the First Fleet Surgeon-General, John White, refer to a sporadic disease (probably gonorrhoea) affecting both marines and those *'who lead irregular lives'*. It involved a *'swelling of the chaps; as that distemper sometimes terminates in ... inflammation of the testicles, so that this complaint ... on the sixth or seventh day, never in one instance failed to fix on those parts'*.

Adding another dimension to the picture, Surgeon-General White described circumstances during the voyage that promoted the spread of STDs among some of the 1350 convicts, sailors and officers aboard the 11 vessel fleet. He reported that the weather *'was now so immoderately hot that the female convicts, perfectly overcome by it, frequently fainted away ... And yet ... so predominant was the warmth of their constitutions or the depravity of their hearts, that the hatches ... could not be suffered to lay off, during the night, without a promiscuous intercourse immediately taking place between them and the seamen and marines.'*

He reported treating some female convicts for *'the venereal'*, a term that entered the English language in the 17th Century to describe the discomfort associated with the exuberant love-making activities attributed to Venus, the goddess of love.

On arrival at Botany Bay, there was ample opportunity for further spread of STDs. Surgeon Arthur Bowes-Smyth reported that *'The men convicts got to them* (the women convicts) *very soon after they landed, and it is beyond my abilities to give a just description of the scene of debauchery and riot that ensued during the night.'*

These and subsequent sexual adventures, helped propel STDs up the league ladder of common medical complaints such that in the

23

early decades of white settlement, they were second only to dysentery.

The impact of STD-associated illness and death on the Aboriginal population has never been fully documented but what evidence there is suggests it was disastrous.

Learning from the past

From time to time in this chapter, mention is made of earlier generations' attitudes and behaviour in the areas of sexual relationships, STDs, prevention and treatments. Examples from the past can help explain why things are the way they are, telling us much about the roots of current attitudes.

Although STDs were widespread in the young colony, discussion of them was an exercise in camouflage. '*Diseases of men and women*' were typically referred to as '*French gout,*' '*ladies fever*', '*errors*', '*contagious sores and blood diseases*' and '*discharges*' for which '*private pills*' could be purchased.

In line with the social norms and morality of the day, authority figures like medical practitioners and parliamentarians tended to bypass frank discussion of the subject. Doctors usually referred to STDs as '*a special illness*', '*a blood disease*', '*a preventable disease*', '*a secret disease*' or a '*vice disease*'. When a law aimed at controlling STDs was discussed in the Queensland Parliament in 1868, members beat around the bush, discussing the subject as one they '*hardly liked to say much about*'.

This would not have mattered much if everyone understood the double-talk associated with sexually acquired infections and if the denial of STDs did not magnify the shame, isolation, fear and widespread ignorance of sufferers, providing fertile breeding grounds for myths and misconceptions.

The failure to discuss STDs in an open way in 19th and early 20th Century Australia threw sufferers burdened by troublesome symptoms and guilty secrets into the arms of quacks who promised quick cures from mail-order manuals and worthless devices. Lack of communication promoted ignorance, medical complications, unintentional disease spread and adverse psychological consequences. Those who found their way into the hospital system had to negotiate a path through a mix of medicine and morality in keeping with the times. By the 1870s, syphilis and gonorrhoea accounted for a significant proportion of patients treated by hospitals. At the Royal Melbourne Hospital, for example, one in every five outpatients seen was an STD sufferer. Those with gonorrhoea had small red discs attached to their cards so they could be segregated from the other patients. At the end of the day's work they were ushered into dingy, cramped quarters to have their mixtures repeated. A history of the hospital reports that these patients *were looked upon as a necessary evil, and little time was wasted in their treatment*. Some hospitals seem to have retained this attitude even to this day.

Church authorities were also involved in the ideological struggle between those who saw the fight against STDs as a battle for sexual morality and those who saw it mainly as a medical problem. To some crusading church leaders, the very suggestion that prophylactic kits should be distributed to soldiers was seen as condoning sexual immorality.

Attempts to improve facilities for treating STDs in Australia were stifled until late in the First World War when it became impossible to ignore the issue any longer. Wars tend to make STDs visible as the need to mobilise a large and healthy armed force brings such illnesses to the forefront of public policy discussions.

In recent decades, the tide has swung towards the view that activities aimed at STD prevention and treatment should focus on campaigns **against** disease, not campaigns **for** sexual morality.

There has also been a gradual shift towards more humane attitudes to people with STDs, accompanied by research and community education about causes, mechanisms of spread and methods of prevention and treatment. This has contributed to a less fearful and defensive attitude to STDs and more open discussion about them.

Social and behavioural barriers to effective action against STDs

Despite some improvements, many obstacles remain to STD prevention, treatment and education, including the following:

Pockets of hostility. When hearing that someone has acquired an STD there is still a widespread tendency to snigger knowingly or use labels like promiscuous, immature, oversexed and permissive.

Such reactions are upsetting and uncaring and raise barriers to treatment-seeking.

Problems with assertiveness. 'It's OK to say no' is one message applicable to people of all ages that is not repeated often enough or loudly enough. Only you know if you are ready to become sexually intimate and only you can take ultimate responsibility for your actions. If you do decide the time is right, it can be difficult to insist on condom use. *'I don't fool around, so I know there's nothing to worry about'* is a standard response to which you have every right to respond in turn, 'If it's not on—it's not on!'

Information is power in this situation and you need to explain clearly and carefully why you believe that every Tom, Jenny and Dick needs protection. If, after a full and fair attempt to explain your views a partner refuses to agree to a condom, it may indicate a lack of regard for you. Respect your partner's opinion but make it clear that what is appropriate for him or her is not acceptable to you in this case. Ultimately no one has as big an interest in your own health as you have yourself. Don't rely on others to take precautions or the law to somehow protect you. Partners may be uninformed, selfish, careless, afraid to be honest, forgetful or they may assume that you have taken protective action.

Difficulties telling partners. If you have an STD, you may worry that an existing or new partner will reject you if you reveal the situation. You may feel 'contaminated' yet be desperately in need of a caring relationship. You may want to tell a partner yet be tempted to put your own needs first. This approach is short-sighted because if the relationship develops, partners inevitably find out and your failure to discuss the situation may result in an irretrievable loss of trust. Sometimes it is only after discussion with 'outsiders', not involved in the relationship, that disclosure begins to seem possible.

On the other hand, your partner may be reluctant to be open with you. He or she may have had one or many partners in the past or may be involved in relationships you know nothing about. Some cultures have strong views about what is acceptable or unacceptable in sexual relationships and these views may work against honesty and the spread of accurate information. The help of a knowledgeable outsider in such situations can be a turning point.

Pressure from others. Safe sex may be considered unfashionable in some groups although this situation in changing with growing awareness of the risks of unprotected sex. It takes courage and maturity to state unpopular views but you may be surprised to find that others feel as you do and were waiting for someone to make the first move.

Feelings of invulnerability. Many young (and older) people associate youth with health and this may lead them to underestimate the risks involved in a particular sexual relationship.

Condom acceptability or availability. Condoms provide significant protection against STDs but there are a number of reasons why some people find them difficult to accept. Practical reasons for resisting their use include their capacity to interfere with lovemaking and their failure to prevent pregnancy or STD transmission if used incorrectly or inconsistently. To be effective, condoms must be rolled onto the erect penis before sex and remain in place until ejaculation. After sex, withdraw the penis, holding the condom firmly to stop any spillage. Point the penis downwards and carefully slip the condom off. Certain religious groups (such as the Roman Catholic Church) frown upon condoms because they are opposed to any form of contraception and because they view their use as an endorsement of casual and multi-partner sex. The opposing view is that condoms are often used by partners in long-term, loving relationships and if people plan to be sexually active, at least they ought to have some protection against infection (and against unintended pregnancy). If you do not have access to a condom when decision time comes, think laterally. There are lots of ways to demonstrate loving feelings that don't put health at risk.

Access to STD diagnostic and treatment services. The reactions of people who suspect they have an STD vary markedly. Some want to obtain a diagnosis quickly and to get prompt treatment. Others try not to think about it, hoping that symptoms will go away. Unfortunately, the longer infections are left untreated, the greater the chance of serious damage and of missing out on treatments that may be effective in the early stages of a disease. Having decided to seek a diagnosis and treatment, telephone your nearest sexual health centre, STD clinic, family planning centre or community health centre for details of the nearest clinic or practitioner

---

Mark is a 24 year-old gay man whose main aim in life is to settle down and live happily with a loving boyfriend. One night he met Peter at a party. They talked a lot and were obviously very attracted to each other. They swapped addresses and agreed to meet for dinner a few days later.

Dinner was very romantic and Mark knew this was going to be the big relationship. Afterwards, Mark and Peter felt so confident about their feelings for each other that they decided to have sex. However Mark was disappointed at Peter's insistence on using a condom. How could such a romantic occasion be spoiled in this way? Why did Peter need a condom—he seemed so healthy, confident and successful? Did Peter think there was something wrong with Mark? Or was he promiscuous?

The next morning, Mark felt somewhat uncertain and Peter guessed he might be anxious about the matter of the condom. Peter wondered how realistic Mark was about the risks involved in unprotected sex. Did Mark allow ideas of romance or judgements about who seemed to be infected interfere with safety? For his part, Peter had tested negative for HIV some months earlier and always used a condom.

---

specialising in STDs. Remember that test results indicating you do not have an STD provide no protection for the future and continued precautions are necessary to protect your health.

The psychological burden of STDs

The diagnosis of an STD may cause problems for the continuation of an existing sexual relationship or for development of new relationships. This may be the result of anger about being infected, fear of rejection, or concern about the possibility of transmitting the infection.

Some people distance themselves from those they love and avoid developing close relationships for many years. In such cases, help is needed to deal with underlying issues such as guilt, anger towards an ex-partner or themselves, and inability to accept that they have an STD.

If and when such individuals resume or start sexual relationships, they may find sexual intimacy nerve-wracking. Fear of passing on an infection or of becoming infected again may be so strong that they don't enjoy the experience. In such situations the use of condoms, even when symptom-free, may be advisable if it enhances feelings of security.

Some people become very depressed, or even suicidal when they learn the diagnosis. They feel that life is over and they will never be able to have a sexual relationship again. Counsellors emphasise that many STDs are manageable, that sufferers can lead a normal life and that self-acceptance is an important part of coping. They also point out that there are many health factors, apart from STDs, that can influence the pleasure derived from sexual relationships. These include prostate troubles, prolapse and menopause-related symptoms such as dryness of the vagina. As with STDs, attention to these problems can bring lasting benefits.

Changing patterns of STD spread

Opportunities for STD transmission remain plentiful. The number of years before partners make commitments to relationships is on the increase, although 'one night stands' seem less common. There is compelling evidence from studies of human sexual behaviour that most men and women have more than one sexual partner in a lifetime, and men are likely to have more partners than women on average.

STDs tend to benefit from such trends because each sexually active person can potentially retain infections (apparent or symptomless), acquired from each of his or her previous sexual partners, who may in turn have acquired infections from any of their partners.

Assessing your STD risk

STDs are not randomly distributed throughout the community. Those at most risk for STDs tend to be involved in behaviour that increases the probability of unprotected exposure to an infected person. The precise estimate of individual risk depends on factors including some or all of the following:

The number of partners you have in a given time. Unless you are using protective measures, the more sexual partners you have

Susie was 17 and madly in love with Michael.

True, he was 25 and her parents did not approve because of his reputation, but when his brown eyes met hers, Susie melted. One weekend they had sex after discussing it previously at length. It was the first time for Susie and a memorable occasion.

A few days later, she noticed a yellow vaginal discharge and a burning sensation when passing urine. Although very concerned, she did not feel able to discuss the matter with her GP who also looked after her parents and brother. The next day the discharge seemed more profuse and she took her courage in both hands and visited a Family Planning Clinic. The doctor explained that an examination and tests were necessary to exclude sexually transmitted diseases and took samples from Susie's vagina and from the urethra, the opening of the bladder.

When Michael saw Susie the next day he suggested they have sex again but she explained she was too sore and wanted to find out what was wrong.

Shortly after, her test results came back positive for both gonorrhoea and for chlamydia. She agreed to have a course of antibiotic tablets. The doctor also impressed on her the importance of returning in three weeks to make sure there was no sign of infection and, in a couple of months, to have a blood test.

or the more partners that your partner has or had previously, the greater is your risk of infection. Selecting partners who are virgins is not a new defence against STDs. Sexual intercourse with somebody *virgo intacta* is perceived to be some sort of guarantee of safety. Tragically, the very people who seek out virgins to protect themselves are often putting others at risk of STDs.

The number and nature of sexual activities you engage in (for instance, oral, anal or vaginal sex).

Your use of protective measures (such as condoms, spermicides, diaphragms).

The chance that your partner has an STD (which in turn depends on his/her risk-taking behaviour and the availability of treatment).

The prevalence of STDs in the population in which partners mix

Health care behaviour, such as whether early attempts are made to get treatment (which may reduce the period of infectiousness).

Your method of contraception. There is an increased risk of STD spread into the Fallopian tubes of women if they use IUDs (Intra Uterine Devices) for contraception. This is a major cause of recurrent abdominal pain and infertility in females and of increased risk of ectopic pregnancy (a pregnancy that develops in the Fallopian tube rather than the uterus). The Pill and Mini Pill appear to provide some protection against such infections but their use may aggravate recurrent thrush.

Trends in the common STDs

More than twenty potentially harmful organisms are spread by sexual contact. Some such as *Chlamydia trachomatis*, genital herpes and the AIDS virus (HIV), are replacing the once-common bacterial STDs such as syphilis, gonorrhoea and chancroid in importance and frequency. These newcomers, regarded as the second generation of STDs, are frequently more difficult to identify, treat and control and can cause particularly serious complications resulting in chronic ill health, disability or death.

Since many STDs do not produce symptoms or are associated with a powerful negative stigma, many cases go unreported. The available information on trends in the occurrence of particular STDs in recent years is discussed in the relevant chapters that follow.

Several high risk groups have been identified but it is important to understand that not all members of such groups are at increased risk and that it is far more informative to talk about high risk behaviours. For most STDs, the age groups at greatest risk are the 20–29 year olds, followed by the 15–19 year age group.

The overall rate of STDs is lower for women than for men and STDs tend to occur at earlier ages in women than men. Some STDs are more common in homosexual men than in heterosexuals. Another group at increased risk of STDs is travellers who go overseas and have sex. In Australia, prostitutes have become very committed to safe sex and, as a result, rates of infection with STDs have decreased in this group in recent years.

The economic impact of STDs

The cost of the community of STDs and their treatment is a matter of increasing relevance as health dollars become more scarce. Costing studies to date have focussed on AIDS.

Few attempts have been made to cost the prevention, diagnosis and treatment of other STDs, the most serious consequences of which tend to affect women and children. For example, a significant proportion of pelvic inflammatory disease (abbreviated as PID, see Chapter 9) is either caused by, or associated with STDs, with consequences including female infertility, ectopic pregnancy and persistent adominal pain. Associated social, psychological and economic costs are considerable and include hospitalisations, surgical procedures, outpatient visits, drug treatments, and disruption of the work and home environment.

As well as ill-health related to PID, there are other important consequences of STDs. Cervical cancer associated with human papilloma virus infection, causes significant illness and many deaths. It costs a substantial amount to screen for HPV-associated cervical abnormalities and to treat them. This is also true of chlamydia, syphilis, gonorrhoea and herpes infection in mothers and their newborn babies.

Chapter Four

SPRINGING LEAKS—GENITAL DISCHARGES: CHLAMYDIA, GONORRHOEA, TRICHOMONAS, CANDIDA, GARDNERELLA

Fluid or pus coming from the eye of the penis (urethral discharge) or from the vagina (vaginal or cervical discharge) are probably the best known symptoms of sexually transmitted disease. However, while well known, a number of special problems can confuse the picture and lead to incorrect treatment.

The first problem is that symptoms may well be much more subtle than is usually realised. In the classic case, males complain of pain on urination (passing pins and needles or dysuria) and a white discharge from the eye of the penis, and females of fluid leaking from the vagina. However, it is now recognised that most infections are usually not so obvious though the complications can be just as serious. Most importantly, in both males and females infections are often symptom free and can go unnoticed.

The second problem is that many people do not clearly understand the important difference between discharges coming from the vagina and discharges that start at the cervix. The organisms that cause cervical discharge are entirely different from those that lead to vaginal discharges. Although these discharges both end up leaking from the opening of the vagina (and are therefore easy to confuse) recognising their difference is the key to diagnosis and treatment.

The third problem is that tests for these various discharges are not perfect and have special requirements to yield accurate and useful results. Specimens can be difficult to obtain, must be taken from the correct place using special procedures, must be sent to the laboratory with special transport arrangements and must be processed with special tests. Specimens for chlamydia testing are difficult to obtain and tests are technically difficult to perform and prone to under or overdiagnosing infections (false positive and false negative results). Therefore results should be interpreted cautiously

33

and only ever in the context of a detailed history and relevant examination findings. How to sort out these problems will be outlined in more detail below.

Discharges from the cervix in women and the eye of the penis in men—Chlamydia and Gonorrhoeae

Unlike vaginal and cervical infections both of which have very different causes and require different approaches, infections of the female cervix and the male urethra are basically due to the same organisms and the treatment approach is similar. The main organisms causing **urethritis** and **cervicitis** are chlamydia (*Chlamydia trachomatis*) and gonorrhoeae (*Neisseria gonorrhoeae*).

John had been involved in many relationships and when he met Linda, they ended up having sex. Because Linda seemed 'clean', he took the condom out of her hand just as she was about to put it on him.

About a week later, John developed a thick yellow discharge from the end of his penis and found passing urine was very uncomfortable. He went to his local doctor who took a sample and examined it under a microscope. Within a few minutes, the doctor was able to tell John he had gonorrhoea. He gave him a prescription for some tablets and explained that this treatment would cure the infection if he took the full course.

John was furious with Linda and determined to 'have it out with her'. They argued about where the blame lay and Linda pointed out that it was she who was ready to apply the condom when John stopped her.

The relationship broke up and John felt sorry for himself. He couldn't believe his bad luck. Why did he always end up hurt? Why were these types of women always attracted to him?

Urethritis is inflammation of the urethra, the tube that drains urine out of the bladder. At its worst, urethritis causes a profuse discharge of pus from the opening and pain on urination. The pain can vary in severity but at its worst has been described as 'like passing razor blades'. More often, however, the symptoms or urethritis are much more subtle. In males, instead of an obvious discharge, the infection may simply cause a slight, clear, sticky leak or a continual moistness under the foreskin or leave small discharge stains on the underpants. Instead of pain on urination, the infection may cause tingling in the eye of the penis (urethral opening or urethral meatus) or tickling along the shaft of the penis under the skin following the line where the urethra runs.

It is often possible to tell the difference between **chlamydia** and **gonorrhoea** just by the pattern of symptoms and signs. Urethritis caused by gonorrhoea is often more profuse and creamier, whereas that caused by chlamydia is usually less severe, the discharge clearer and less in volume and less uncomfortable. However, it must be emphasised that both infections can be symptom free and sometimes chlamydia can be severe enough to lead to an initial diagnosis of suspected gonorrhoea. Furthermore, various studies have recognised that up to 35% of men with gonorrhoea also have a concurrent chlamydia infection. This provides the basis for the normal practice of prescribing a treatment for gonorrhoea that also treats chlamydia.

Cervicitis is inflammation of the female cervix (the entrance to the uterus or womb at the top end of the vagina). Because the cervix is hidden in the body there are usually very few symptoms, if any, and the infection is often first noted because the sexual partner develops symptoms, or signs of infection are found during routine examination or on a routine test such as a Pap smear. A common problem occurs when one partner has an infection diagnosed but the other partner(s) fails to get treated. This may be because contact has been lost, or a person is too afraid or too embarrassed to inform any partners. Another common problem occurs when the health worker neglects to inform the patient of the importance of arranging treatment or where the partner attends for a checkup and nothing is found. With subtle symptoms and imperfect tests, if one person has a proven infection then his or her partner must be treated regardless of what is found during a checkup.

If left untreated, both gonorrhoea and chlamydia can lead to serious complications in both men and women. Either can migrate further along the genital tract and cause deep inflammation. In women this is called **pelvic inflammatory disease (PID)**, in men the equivalent is **epididymo-orchitis** and **prostatitis**. Because the principles are very similar these probably should be called **male PID**.

Seven weeks ago Nerita had her first-ever experience of sex with her boyfriend, Brad, with whom she had been going out for a year. Then last week she woke with cramps in her lower abdomen and had a slight fever.

She saw her local doctor who found a slight discharge seeping from her cervix. There was also tenderness in the lower right part of her pelvis (the iliac fossa). The doctor examined a sample of the discharge under a microscope and found pus, but no evidence of gonorrhoea. She wondered if Nerita had pelvic inflammatory disease due to chlamydia.

Because the pain was more severe on one side, the doctor also did a test to check if Nerita had an ectopic pregnancy (that is, a pregnancy that grows inside the Fallopian tube instead of in the uterus). The pregnancy test was negative and Nerita started a course of antibiotics to treat the pelvic inflammatory disease. The doctor also asked to see Brad, and took a sample for testing from the eye of his penis. She prescribed him antibiotics although he did not have any symptoms.

Today, the chlamydia culture results came through; Brad's was positive, and Nerita's negative. When giving the results, the doctor reminded the couple about the importance of completing their antibiotics.

The symptoms of PID in women include deep pelvic pain and, sometimes, fever. Untreated, these symptoms can go through cycles of silence and flare-up. Often the pelvic infection can silently and gradually damage a woman's Fallopian tubes, the ducts that carry the egg from the ovaries to the uterus. If these are damaged, a woman can become infertile or, if she does become pregnant, there is a greater chance that the fertilised egg (embryo) will become lodged in an abnormal Fallopian tube. This is known as an ectopic pregnancy and can result in serious, often life threatening complications. In the early stages of PID, the infection can be treated and the damage is reversible. At later stages, the damage is very difficult to reverse and pregnancy may need to be assisted with in-vitro fertilisation (IVF or test tube baby program). Many medical practitioners believe that women with PID should be given prolonged antibiotic treatment. There seems to be no clear agreement on how long treatment should continue, but it is not unusual for antibiotics to be prescribed for four to six weeks.

Epididymo-orchitis is the name given to an infection involving the testes and the tubes connected to the testes (the epididymis). The infection can cause pain and aching and it is usually possible to feel a tender swelling just behind the testicle (in the epididymis). Again, if the infection is left untreated for a prolonged period of time, the damage can lead to decreased fertility. This is not as well understood in men as it is in women. The most likely cause of severe problems is untreated gonorrhoea infection, an uncommon occurrence in most Western countries. There is evidence that decreased fertility can result from silent chlamydia infection.

In addition to infection of the Fallopian tubes and epididymis, chlamydia can also occasionally spread to other areas. In women it can leave the pelvis and infect the outside of the liver. This is called the Fitz-Hugh-Curtis syndrome and although it sounds serious, it is usually very mild and easily treated. In men some infections can also spread to the prostate gland and cause prostatitis. This syndrome can cause fever and a chronic ache between the base of the penis and the rectum. Prostatitis is notoriously difficult to treat and usually requires prolonged treatment with antibiotics (such as doxycycline and/or ciprofloxacin). Occasionally after entering the bloodstream, gonorrhoea can spread to the joints and cause joint infection (septic arthritis), or to the heart valves (endocarditis).

Treatment of gonorrhoea and chlamydia

Most species of gonorrhoea are sensitive to penicillin-derivatives and are best eradicated by a single high dose, usually given by injection. A drug called probenecid can be given half an hour beforehand which slows the excretion of penicillin making it more effective. For people allergic to penicillin, ciprofloxacin is usually given.

There are some species of gonorrhoea which have the ability to make a substance that inactivates penicillins and they are therefore resistant to this therapy. It is therefore essential that drug sensitivity of the organism is established, and that an appropriate antibiotic is given.

The treatment of chlamydia involves using one of the groups of tetracyclines, especially doxycycline. These are usually administered for ten to fourteen days or occasionally, when PID also occurs, for up to four weeks.

Traps in diagnosing and managing chlamydia and gonorrhoea

Tests for chlamydia and gonorrhoea have a number of idiosyncracies that can confuse the diagnosis.

The key to testing for these infections in men is to take a sample of the discharge and smear it onto a glass microscope slide. The smear is then stained and examined under the microscope. This is known as a gram stain. If the sample is properly taken there should be signs of inflammation (white blood cells called polymorphs). Furthermore, if the inflammation is due to gonorrhoea, then the organisms can usually be seen mixed with the white cells. If white cells but no organisms are seen, then the infection is called **non-specific urethritis (NSU)**. The most common cause of NSU is chlamydia. The gram stain takes five minutes and treatment for gonorrhoea or chlamydia can be started immediately before further results are returned. Cultures for gonorrhoea and chlamydia are also undertaken to confirm the diagnosis and to check that the gonorrhoea will respond to the antibiotics prescribed.

The growth of organisms in the laboratory is known as culture and for both chylamdia and gonorrhoea it can be tricky. Samples should be taken from the eye of the urethra in men and the cervix in women. A sample from the vagina is not appropriate and will not yield the organism. The gonorrhoea specimen should be put on a special charcoal-coated swab or placed into a fluid containing charcoal. The charcoal absorbs toxins and helps to keep the gonorrhoea alive until testing can occur. The specimen should be transported to the testing laboratory at room temperature, as refrigeration can kill gonorrhoea. At the laboratory, the organism is tested on a special gonococcal culture plate.

Unlike the gonorrhoea specimen, the chlamydia specimen should not be pus or discharge. Chlamydia lives in the cells lining the

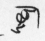

urethra and the cervix. The discharge should be wiped away when the gonorrhoea swab is taken and then the fine chlamydia swab should be gently inserted into the urethra or vagina and carefully rotated in order to collect some of the cells lining the urethra or the cervix. While this sounds uncomfortable, if done carefully, it is usually not a problem. The chlamydia swab is then placed into a fluid especially designed to keep chlamydia alive while in transit to the laboratory. Unlike the gonorrhoea specimen, this specimen should be kept cold but not frozen. If the specimen is frozen or if the specimen is warm, the organism will die more quickly and culture will fail. Deep infections causing female or male PID may not give positive results because the infection may no longer be present in the urethra or the cervix.

As can be seen, there are a number of points at which problems can occur and the diagnosis can be missed.

In an attempt to overcome some of these difficulties, new tests to detect chlamydia have been introduced. These are called immunofluorescence (IF) and ELISA tests. They rely on detecting surface components of the chlamydia, called antigens, and they do not require the chlamydia to arrive in the laboratory alive. Unfortunately, while these tests are useful, they have not met expectations and can result in false positive and false negative results. False negative means that the person has the infection but the test has failed to detect it. False positive means that the person does not have the infection but the test result incorrectly says that he or she does. The serious implications for a relationship of an incorrect diagnosis are obvious. Nevertheless, these tests are commonly used to diagnose chlamydia. Hence results must be interpreted with care. The only way to prove a chlamydia infection is present is with a positive chlamydia culture. Because of the long term consequences, a doctor may recommend treatment for an infection even if the evidence for its presence is weak.

Both chlamydia and gonorrhoea can cause infections in places other than the cervix and urethra. This includes the moist surfaces of the throat, the rectum and the eye. Infections of the throat and rectum are usually symptom free, although occasionally there can be a rectal discharge particularly with gonorrhoea. Eye infections can be mild, in the case of chlamydia and very severe with gonorrhoea. These infections are passed on by direct contact with the infected secretions. Therefore, for example, both gonorrhoea and chlamydia can be passed on through oral sex. Babies born to mothers with untreated infection can pick up chlamydia or gonorrhoea during birth. Gonorrhoea in the baby's eye can cause a severe infection that can rapidly lead to blindness. To prevent this the mother can be tested and treated prior to giving birth or, failing that, the baby can be treated as soon as possible after birth. Chlamydia can cause a milder infection in babies that can be treated with an antibiotic called erythromycin. If untreated, chlamydia can also cause pneumonia in newborn babies.

Sometimes urethritis proves very difficult to treat and occasionally other organisms have been shown to cause urethritis. These should be suspected particularly when treatment has failed. A doctor should always open up the opening of the urethra (the meatus) and check for a meatal wart. Occasionally, people can have a solitary wart just inside the urethral opening which can cause recurring symptoms. Warts do not respond to antibiotics and symptoms probably won't clear until the wart has been specifically treated. Herpes can also cause a symptom pattern similar to urethritis. Again, if antibiotics do not seem to be successful, a sample should be taken from inside the opening and sent to a pathology laboratory for herpes viral culture. Ureaplasmas and trichomonas can also cause urethritis in males on occasion. Drugs that are active against chlamydia should also work against ureaplasma but metronidazole will be necessary to treat trichomonas.

Apart from the infections mentioned above, there is considerable disagreement as to what causes persistent non-specific urethritis. In the absence of any other findings, most doctors will stop treating the problem after three courses of antibiotics even if mild symptoms continue. Typically, the antibiotics include two courses of doxycycline and one course of erythromycin and metronidazole. It is important to take the antibiotics conscientiously, and to let the doctor know if there has been any diarrhoea, vomiting or other reason for the antibiotics to be ineffective. As usual, it is important to ensure that the regular partner has also been properly treated. It is generally felt that any sexually transmitted cause of urethritis will be cured with this treatment and that any residual symptoms are either due to some unimportant organism or to a continuing inflammation after the infection has been dealt with. The symptoms will eventually resolve.

After a record-breaking season with his local football team, Peter was looking forward to the end of year trip. The Gold Coast hotel where the team stayed was within a short distance of a well-known disco and, in no time at all, Peter had teamed up with a brunette. By midnight Peter and the brunette had retired to his room where some adventurous sex followed.

About ten days after returning home to his wife and family, he woke up one morning with a very sore right testicle. When he tried to urinate, it was like passing pins and needles. He rang his doctor who was able to see him promptly and who examined his very sore and swollen testicle as well as his urinary system.

The doctor raised the possibility of a sexually transmitted disease after completing the examination and hearing about the Gold Coast trip. He referred Peter to an STD clinic where the doctor passed a small cotton wool swab into Peter's penis and, after examination by a pathologist, relayed the diagnosis of gonorrhoea.

The doctor prescribed a course of antibiotic capsules, organised a follow-up appointment for Peter, and endeavoured to explain how essential it was that his wife, and any other sexual partner, also be treated.

Vaginal discharges

As noted previously, vaginal discharges are due to a different and diverse group of organisms to those that cause cervical infections and they require different tests and treatments. Indeed, many vaginal discharges are not even sexually transmitted. It is normal for the vagina to be moist and, at different times during a cycle, the normal vaginal secretions may become thicker or increase in amount. One of the keys to distinguishing a normal vaginal discharge from an abnormal one is whether the discharge differs from what is normal for a particular woman. Examination, a Pap smear and a gram stain can be helpful.

Vaginal discharges due to infections include those caused by *candida* (a fungus), *gardnerella* (a bacterium), *trichomonas* (a protozoan) and sometimes even *herpes* (a virus).

Candida, also called thrush, is normally present in the intestine and can often also be found in the vagina without causing any symptoms. Thrush is not normally sexually transmitted and usually causes a problem only when vaginal conditions permit. Factors that favour candida becoming a problem are reduced immunity, the removal of normal, competing bacteria and warm, moist conditions. These factors may be present because of diabetes, poor immunity, antibiotics, douching, other discharges, sweating or the wearing of restrictive, hot clothing such as pantyhose, leggings, leather pants, gym gear and tight jeans. Candida typically causes an itching, red infection of the vagina and the labia (vaginal lips). The discharge is white and tends to clump, looking like cottage cheese. Should the infection continue untreated, the itching can cause significant discomfort due mainly to the raw, scratched areas.

Testing for candida is relatively easy. Samples of the discharge can be examined under the microscope and with standard bacterial culture methods. Treatment is with vaginal creams or vaginal tablets (pessaries) containing antifungal medications. Antifungal tablets, such as nystatin, taken by mouth will not treat vaginal thrush because the medication is not absorbed from the intestine into the blood stream and does not reach the vagina. Newer treatments are now being developed that can be taken by mouth (e.g. fluconazole) but these are usually reserved for cases that won't respond to more simple treatments.

Attention also needs to be directed towards correcting the underlying reasons why candida has become a problem. Treating diabetes, wearing loose airy clothing and only using antibiotics when there are good reasons, all help. In women prone to repeated thrush, antibiotics in the form of vaginal pessaries or cream are appropriate. In extreme cases, some practitioners will resort to treating both partners with local creams and tablets by mouth in an attempt to eradicate the organism totally. This is rarely necessary and unlikely to cause a permanent resolution. The intestines of both partners will probably become inhabited with candida again fairly quickly.

Gardnerella is a bacterium which typically causes a smelly discharge. There is usually no irritation or itch but examination of the vagina usually shows a greyish sticky discharge that smells 'fishy'. Gardneralla is basically a problem of an imbalance of the vaginal environment. This imbalance causes the normal, harmless lactobacilli to disappear and allows organisms including gardnerella

Cal, aged 25, recently holidayed in the Pacific islands and on returning home, noticed small itchy red spots on the head of his penis.

Cal tried to ignore them because he did not want his private parts examined by a doctor. But over the following days, the spots became redder and itchier. He also noticed a white paste collecting under his foreskin and a raw feeling around the head of his penis. After an attack of anxiety, he plucked up courage and saw his local doctor who diagnosed thrush under the foreskin.

This was easily treated with a cream used for tinea. The doctor did not check for any sexually transmitted infections because Cal had never had sex.

The doctor took the opportunity to reassure Cal and to advise him about sexual safety. He gave Cal some condoms and lubricant to practise with at home so that if he ever did decide to have sex, he could do so safely.

to multiply to abnormal levels in conjunction with other organisms called anaerobes. The anaerobes probably cause the smell.

The infection can be confirmed by examining a sample of the discharge under the microscope with a gram stain. Usually the gram stain demonstrates 'clue' cells. These are vaginal cells that are coated with bacteria. Some practitioners also check the acidity (pH) of the vagina. This is because gardnerella is a disturbance of the vaginal environment and the vagina becomes much less acidic. Vaginal pH is usually less than 4.5. In gardnerella it is usually greater than 5.5. Some doctors even do the 'whiff' test. In this test, a small sample of the discharge is placed on a glass microscope slide and a drop of potassium hydroxide (10% KOH) is added. This intensifies the 'fishy' smell and makes the diagnosis easier.

Treatment is designed to reduce the overpopulation of the vagina with gardnerella and anaerobes and to restore the normal, harmless, protective bacteria (lactobacilli). Some people have tried to do this with yoghurt. Yoghurt is acidic and is fermented with lactobacilli similar, but not identical, to those in the vagina. Yoghurt is put in the vagina in an attempt to restore the balance. Some people prefer a more 'medical' version of this called 'Acigel'. This is simply an acidifying jelly. Other people prefer to take antibiotics, particularly if the infection is not responding well to the other treatments. Amoxicillin and metronidazole are often used. Treatment of gardnerella is also directed towards correcting the underlying cause of the vaginal disturbance. Douching, vaginal deodorants and forgotten tampons may all contribute.

Meherun was shy, but lately she had become more withdrawn and had not left the house for eight days. In desperation, her mother decided to take her to the local doctor in order to get a referral to a psychiatrist.

The doctor spent a long time talking to Meherun and eventually found that she was worried about a foul-smelling vaginal discharge. After lots of explanation and talking, Meherun asked the doctor for a careful examination. This revealed no sign of inflammation or abnormality, but a thick grey-green discharge with a fishy smell was evident. After examining the sample under a microscope, the doctor quickly concluded the problem was gardnerella.

Meherun had never had sex and was relieved to know that everything was in order apart from the infection. The bacterial vaginosis was treated easily with metronidazole and all other tests were normal. Meherun's mood lifted and she was happier and more confident from then on.

Trichomonas is a protozoan. These are larger and more 'advanced' organisms than bacteria but are still microscopic. The way that trichomonas spreads is not entirely clear but it is likely that most infections are sexually transmitted. The typical pattern of trichomonas is of an irritating vaginal discharge. Examination usually reveals red vaginal surfaces and a 'frothy' discharge. Sometimes, the cervix has a red spotted appearance and is called a 'strawberry' cervix. In men, trichomonas can occasionally produce symptoms. These include slight discomfort when passing urine. Trichomonas is easy to diagnose. A sample of the discharge is taken and placed on a microscope slide and examined while it is still wet. The 'trich' can usually be seen swimming erratically around. Treatment is with antibiotics: metronidazole or tinidazole.

Herpes can occasionally cause a vaginal discharge. This is most

Ingrid, a sex worker for the last three years, knows a lot about HIV and always uses condoms at work. She is very skilled and can even put condoms on customers without them being aware of it. She has a medical check every month and has never had a sexually transmitted infection.

Ingrid also has a private life and a new boyfriend, Karl, who has a mental block about using condoms (he says he loses his erection). One night, Ingrid agreed to have unprotected intercourse with Karl and a week later, she felt a slight burning around the vulva. She also seemed to have more moisture than usual coming from the vagina and this watery fluid had a slight 'fishy' smell.

She took Karl along with her to her regular medical check which revealed she had a trichomonas infection. A sample from Karl also showed trichomonas, although he had no symptoms. Both were treated and all other tests were negative.

Now Karl has problems keeping his erection unless he uses a condom!

likely in the first episode of herpes. The discharge comes from herpes ulcers usually high in the vagina and the outer part of the cervix (ectocervix). Sometimes, a clear discharge from the surface of the ulcers is fairly profuse. Usually, however, painful ulcers are the most prominent sign of herpes. When a doctor is in doubt, a herpes culture should be performed. Herpes is discussed in more detail in the chapter on genital ulcers.

Special note—confusing urinary problems with sexually transmitted infections

Occasionally, a vaginal discharge is confused with mild **loss of bladder control**. A doctor can usually clarify the situation by investigating the pattern of the problem and by performing an examination. Bladder control problems tend to occur in women in late-middle age who have had a number of children. Affected women may also have recently noticed a lump in the vagina. The main problem is a stretching and weakening of the pelvic muscles.

Monica visited her doctor three times within four weeks complaining of an itchy, smelly vaginal discharge.

On the first and second occasions, the doctor checked the interior of Monica's vagina, commented that the creamy discharge was probably due to thrush and prescribed a vaginal cream and vaginal tablets. These provided some relief but the discharge did not disappear and there was a persistent yellow-grey stain on Monica's underwear. All the while, she did not have intercourse in line with her doctor's advice.

When she returned the third time, the doctor decided to sample the discharge. She placed some cotton swabs into Monica's vagina, then sent the swabs for testing.

On Monica's return three days later, the doctor said the organisms were *Gardnerella vaginalis* which would not respond to the anti-fungal treatment prescribed previously for the thrush. She gave Monica four antibiotic tablets to take that evening and another four for her partner, and reassured her that the discharge would probably clear within two or three days.

Within a few days Monica rang the doctor to let her know that both the discharge and the staining had vanished.

If the bladder drops due to the stretching of the pelvic muscles and bulges into the vagina (in Medispeak, a prolapse), the woman will often complain of a lump and difficulty in stopping the bladder from leaking. Often the urine will leak only when pressure is placed on the lower abdomen. This means that control is lost only when the woman coughs, strains or goes up in lifts! Control can sometimes be restored with pelvic muscle exercises, but in many cases surgery is necessary. The problem is clearly not one of infection.

Bladder infections can be confused with gonorrhoea or chlamydia. This is because they can cause pain on urination, discomfort in the lower abdomen and fever. If the infection moves to the kidneys then it can produce pain in the lower back. A bladder infection can be detected by examining a sample of urine under the microscope and by culturing the urine. The sample needs to be a 'mid-stream' specimen, that is, a specimen taken during urination around the time that the bladder is about half empty. Special care must be taken to obtain as clean a specimen as possible. Pubic hairs, lint or vaginal discharge that drop into the specimen will contaminate it and make it difficult to test. The specimen should only be collected in a sterile container.

Bladder infections are not sexually transmitted diseases and they can be easily treated with antibiotics. But the infections can be related to intercourse in some women. This is because in women, the urethra is very short and the movements of intercourse may briefly open up the urethra and allow an infection to enter. In men this is unlikely, and a bladder infection in them suggests that there may be a serious abnormality of the urinary system. Special tests including kidney x-rays need to be performed if no explanation for the infection can be found in men and if repeated infections occur in women.

Conclusion

The differences between cervical and vaginal discharges cannot be over-emphasised. It is a common mistake to lump all discharges together but they may be due to very different infections and require very different tests and treatments. Indeed, most vaginal discharges are usually not sexually transmitted infections.

Cervicitis and urethritis on the other hand, are usually due to either of two organisms; chlamydia and/or gonorrhoea both of which are STDs. The symptoms of these infections can be quite subtle and they are often symptom-free. Untreated, these infections can lead to serious complications. In women, the organism may move to the uterus, the Fallopian tubes and even as far as the liver. Infection in the pelvis can cause pelvic inflammatory disease (PID) and lead to infertility and ectopic pregnancies if left untreated. In men, the infection may spread to cause a painful infection involving the prostate and the epididymis. At these more advanced stages, treatment can be difficult not least because of problems with testing. Test results should not be viewed as infallible. If the clinical pattern is one of infection but the test is negative, it may still be sensible to treat a suspected infection. If the pattern is not suggestive of infection, the decision becomes more difficult. A doctor may decide not to treat if there seems no likely explanation for having an infection and the positive test was unexpected. On the other hand, because infections are often symptom-less and the complications potentially serious, treatment may be advised even without a positive test. In either case the practitioner needs to be acutely aware of the social and psychological implications of the diagnosis and to be as objective as possible in assessing the risk of acquiring a sexually transmitted infection.

Chapter Five

LUMPS, BUMPS, WARTS AND ALL: SWOLLEN GLANDS, GENITAL WARTS, MOLLUSCUM

Warts are small fleshy growths on skin and moist surfaces (mucous membranes). True warts are due to a viral infection known as the *human papilloma virus* or HPV. In addition to typical warts, the wart virus can also cause infection without symptoms or may simply cause a slight thickening of the skin leading to annoying symptoms such as abrasions, cracking and dryness. Obviously, warts are not the only cause of such symptoms.

Over the last few years, some strains of the wart virus have been associated with cancer of the cervix. For some people this can be frightening. A clear explanation is important in order to place this in perspective: the wart virus link is one of a number of factors, a minority of wart virus strains are involved in cervical cancer and, regardless of wart infection, with regular Pap smears, cancer of the cervix is preventable.

Molluscum contageosum is a virus infection of the skin that also causes a wart-like appearance. However, closer examination of a molluscum reveals some particular characteristics that allow it to be distinguished from true warts. It is important to establish the difference between warts and mollusca because Molluscum contageosum does not appear to pose a serious risk to health whereas some wart virus infections may.

Totally different in appearance, but considered within the 'lumps and bumps' section of this book are 'swollen glands', also known as enlarged lymph nodes. Enlarged lymph nodes can occur in response to a number of infections as well as to other problems. Lymph nodes can be swollen where there is local, or more widespread, infection. In the case of infections that involve the entire body, nodes will be enlarged in many places. In the case of local infections, the nodes closest to the site of infection will be enlarged first. In most visible genital infections, this usually means that the inguinal nodes (in the groin, at the top of the leg) will be enlarged. Two difficulties worth noting are firstly that often genital infections do not cause any enlargement of nodes and that secondly, the inguinal lymph nodes are usually easy to feel and are therefore often mistakenly thought of as enlarged.

What's normal—pitfalls for the unwary

There are two primary difficulties associated with warty lesions of the genitals. The first is the occasional difficulty for the inexperienced in distinguishing normal structures from warts. The second is the variety of appearances of wart virus infection. These include warts; low grade infections that cause minor problems without causing warts; and infections that have no symptoms.

It is not unusual for a patient to attend an STD clinic after having had several treatments for wart-like problems that on closer examination are not warts but are normal variations of the skin of the genitals. This is not entirely surprising because there are a number of structures on the skin that can look a little warty! Four structures along the shaft of the penis are particularly prone to being confused with warts or other abnormalities. These are 'pearly penile papules', sebaceous glands, hair follicles and Tyson's glands. It is helpful to be able to recognise these structures in order to avoid pointless anxiety and unnecessary treatment. Often, it is better to get a second opinion from an STD specialist if there is any doubt about whether genital structures are normal or not.

Of the four structures mentioned, perhaps pearly penile papules are most commonly mistaken for warts. These are tiny fleshy tags that run around the edge of the head or 'glans' of the penis just before the head joins the shaft. In about 10% of men, they are particularly prominent and are often a cause for unnecessary concern. The key to their identification is both their location and their fairly regular distribution in rows around the edge of the head of the penis (the corona).

Another cause for unecessary concern in some younger men and women is small hair follicles and sebaceous glands. Hair follicles can appear as tiny raised, whitish spots along the shaft of the penis, on the scrotum and on the vaginal lips (labia). In some areas, the follicles may have no obvious hair protruding from them and look

Geoff, a 16-year-old student in his final school year spent a lot of time studying and was under intense pressure. Unfortunately he did not do as well as expected in his practice exams and his father, noticing that he seemed unhappy and preoccupied, asked if there was anything he could do to help.

Initially, Geoff clammed up but, after a few days, he explained that he was worried sick about some spots he had found on his penis a couple of months earlier.

Geoff went to the local doctor, and his father waited in the waiting room for moral support. The doctor thought he might have genital warts and referred him to an STD clinic for treatment. The STD specialist found a row of tiny spots like 'goose bumps' arranged evenly around the rim of the head of the penis. He explained that these were typical, harmless 'pearly penile papules' and needed no treatment.

Reassured, Geoff was able to apply himself to his final examination without the burden of worry he had been carrying.

very similar to 'goose-bumps'. The clue to their identification is that they are more common on the shaft and towards the base of the penis and scrotum and towards the more hairy areas of the labia and they are fairly evenly scattered. They seem to be lying just under normal skin rather than growing from it as in the case of warts. Needless to say, treatment is not necessary but reassurance and explanation are essential.

Sebaceous glands can also lead to spots and lumps. These glands are normal skin glands that produce substances that keep the skin soft and moisturised. If these glands have no outlet onto the skin or if the gland becomes blocked, the creamy sebaceous material accumulates and forms a round 'pea-like' lump called a cyst. If the cyst becomes infected, it can become red and painful. The cysts are usually found on the more hairy areas of the genitals particularly on the scrotum and outer labia. Sometimes there can be several cysts. Treatment is usually not necessary but antibiotics may be called for if the cyst is infected. Often, simple surgery is required to remove troublesome cysts. Sebaceous glands that are functioning entirely normally are often found in clusters along the underside of the shaft of the penis where they form a prominent collection of white spots. This is a variation on normal.

Tyson's glands are small glands found on either side of the frenulum of the penis (the frenulum is the skin that ties the underside of the head of the penis to the shaft of the penis or to the foreskin). There is usually one gland on either side of the frenulum about 1 mm in diameter. These are usually round and 'pearly' in appearance and are also normal.

Other glands can also become infected and cause painful lumps. For example, Bartholin's glands are located in the bottom end of the vaginal lips (labia). If they become infected (often with gonorrhoea) they can become enlarged and painful. Treatment is with antibiotics but they often also need incising to drain the pus in order for treatment to be effective.

Finally, the remnants of the hymen just inside the entrance of the vagina can sometimes look like skin tags. This appearance is quite normal and should not be confused with warts.

Warts

Although warts have been known through the ages and are the subject of numerous myths, it is only very recently that anything at all has been known about the biology of the wart or *human papilloma* virus. Unlike most other viruses associated with sexually transmitted infections, it is not possible to grow wart virus in the laboratory and this has delayed progress in understanding the virus. Recently, however, it has been possible to study warts using molecular biology methods. Using these methods, it has been found that there are around sixty to eighty different types of wart virus. Of these, types 6, 11 and 16 are commonly found in genital infections. All types of wart virus seem to be able to cause a few or no symptoms and some do not normally infect the genitals. As far as genital infections go, types 6 and 11 are the most common cause of obvious genital warts and types 16 and 18 seem to be a less likely cause of 'classic' warts. On the other hand, types 16, 18 and 31 have been recently linked to cancer of the cervix particularly in conjunction with other factors such as smoking.

The paradox with important counselling implications is, therefore, that women who have had obvious warts may well not be infected with a virus with potentially serious consequences, whereas those who have had no sign of warts may still carry the potentially serious strains of the wart virus. This is reassuring for those who are anxious because they have had genital warts. It also underlines the import- ance of prevention and of regular Pap smears for all women who have had intercourse, regardless of age and regardless of whether warts have been found.

Largely due to improved experimental testing methods, the pattern of wart virus infection is now better understood. It is clear that wart virus infection can have a variety of manifestations. Classic wart infections look like small skin tags, they are usually softer and more moist than warts on other tougher, more dry skin. In new infections they can often be very numerous and multiply rapidly over a couple of weeks. Usually, the warts are most numerous in soft and damp areas such as under the foreskin, around the anus and along the inner lips of the vagina (labia minora). In these situations, they are often whiter than the surrounding skin, firmer and rougher than normal skin to touch, and quite moist. This appearance is sometimes described as a 'cauliflower' appearance. In severe cases, bacteria can lodge among the warts and, if moist, can produce a slight, smelly discharge. After going through this florid, prolific phase, warts then typically enter a phase where they become less numerous and look more like occasional tags of normal-looking skin. In this form they can often persist for several months before disappearing. Treatment speeds this process up.

Wart virus infection can also cause other symptom patterns. Many people with wart virus infection do not develop obvious warts, indeed many have no symptoms at all. Some people develop a mild thickening of the involved skin and the skin can then lose its elasticity and is more likely to become abraded or to crack when stretched. These cracks and abrasions can be tender and may lead patients and doctors to think that herpes is causing the problem despite negative tests. This effect can be even more pronounced if the infection occurs at a site that is continually moist. The place most prone to this sort of problem in men is the frenulum and in women the meeting point of the vaginal lips below the vaginal opening, just in front of the anus.

Warts do not necessarily develop as soon as a person becomes infected. The time between infection and the appearance of warts varies from a couple of weeks to some years. The appearance of warts, therefore, does not necessarily indicate that a partner has been 'unfaithful'. Once developed, warts can persist for periods ranging from a couple of weeks to many months. Some people find them reappearing on and off over some years. In most people, however, there is a period of several weeks of activity and then they progressively disappear. It is not uncommon for people who have had warts to observe that a seemingly minor trauma to a wart is followed by the warts clearing completely. It may be that the trauma was sufficient to stimulate a degree of immunity against warts, thus causing them to disappear. It seems unlikely, however, that the wart virus is ever completely eradicated and probably the infection moves into a more latent phase during which no obvious warts can be found but wart virus can still be detected with special tests in samples of normal looking skin from the previously affected areas. This is exactly what happens when wart virus is detected on a Pap smear even though the person no longer has warts or may never have had them.

Wart virus with a low level of activity can often be detected by using 5% acetic acid (acetic acid is the main component of vinegar) applied to the skin or moist surface for five minutes. This test is most useful during a colposcopy examination. Colposcopy is a detailed examination that should be performed whenever a Pap smear suggests abnormalities such as a precursor of cancer, known as **CIN (Cervical Intraepithelial Neoplasia)**. Colposcopy involves examining the woman's cervix with an instrument called a colposcope. This is a specialised microscope that can be used to look into the vagina towards the cervix during a vaginal examination. Painting the cervix with 5% acetic acid causes most wart-affected areas to become whiter than the surrounding normal moist surfaces and causes most abnormalities to become visible. Once visible, they can be examined under magnification for serious abnormalities using the colposcope. Sometimes it is possible to treat the abnormality at the time of the examination, whereas at other times, a sample of the abnormal tissue may be removed and sent to a pathologist for more accurate diagnosis.

Anxious patients often request a checkup for warts using 5% acetic acid painted onto their genital skin. Whilst this is possible, it is not usually very helpful. Firstly, some areas of wart virus infection do not turn white following the application of acetic acid, whereas some areas of irritation may react without being infected. Secondly, if the other partner is infected and the couple have had intercourse, then it is likely that both have been exposed and that the test will do no more than confirm the infection. Thirdly, current evidence suggests that infection is for life and, whilst warts can be removed, the virus is unlikely to be totally eradicated by treatment and actively seeking out areas of infection is fairly pointless.

Treatment of warts can be complicated. Various methods are used to kill visible warts such as painting with a paint called podophyllin, freezing with liquid nitrogen or dry ice, zapping with an electric current (diathermy) or laser and surgery. These methods generally cause direct damage to warts and in some cases seem to speed up their disappearance possibly by stimulating the immune system. However, this immunity is probably not perfect and even if the warts disappear, there is no evidence that the virus is ever totally eradicated from apparently normal skin. There is also no clear evidence that treatment prevents transfer of the virus, although it does seem that treatment of fresh, active warts reduces the chance that this will occur. Treatment also does not seem to prevent an individual from subsequently contracting other, possibly more serious strains of the wart virus. Treatment is therefore largely a matter of appearance. No matter which form of treatment is used, solitary attempts at treatment never seem to be sufficient to clear the warts. It is important that patients are informed of this in order to prevent them from becoming disillusioned and to encourage them to return for further management.

In summary, treatment of warts:

1. is largely cosmetic
2. is aimed at speeding up the disappearance of warts in their most active phase
3. may act by stimulating local (imperfect) immunity
4. is unlikely to completely remove the virus which will still be carried in a more latent form in apparently normal skin
5. is unlikely to prevent the virus from being passed on
6. will not prevent the person from becoming infected with new strains of wart virus
7. will rarely be successful with one treatment only and will usually need to be repeated several times.

Currently it would seem sensible to treat obvious warts for the sake of appearance, to recommend regular yearly Pap smears for all women and to recommend precautions such as using condoms for new partners.

Domes with dimples: Mollusca

The *Molluscum contageosum* virus is a member of the pox virus family and, despite some superficial similarities, is not related to wart viruses. It is spread by direct contact with infected skin. Because the virus is passed from person to person by such contact, the mollusca have been referred to as 'wrestlers nodules'. The time between contact with the virus and the appearance of mollusca on the skin is between a week and six months (average two to three months). Mollusca appear as warty structures that can usually be distinguished from warts by their characteristic appearance: Mollusca tend to be rounder domes with a dent or 'plug' in the centre called an umbilication. The skin over the dome is often smoother and shinier than normal skin or warty skin. Lifting the 'plug' and then gently squeezing will often cause a small amount of creamy material to be pushed out from the centre. It has been proposed that this material originates from the centre of the molluscum where the virus is most active and that it may be this material that is able to spread the virus.

Conclusion

There are a number of normal structures that can be mistaken for abnormalities of the penis and female genitals.

Genital wart virus can have a variety of appearances ranging from typical warts, to skin thickening and irritation, to an infection with no obvious abnormality. Only a few of about sixty strains of wart virus have been associated with cancer of the cervix (see Chapter 9). These strains may never cause warts. Paradoxically, people who have had warts may not have the virus linked to this cancer, whereas people can be infected with the more serious strains and yet show no sign of warts. Pap smears are essential for all women who have had intercourse: cancer of the cervix should be a preventable disease.

Chapter Six

BLISTERS, ULCERS, ABRASIONS, RAW AREAS AND SCABS: HERPES, EARLY SYPHILIS, CHANCROID, DONOVANOSIS, TRAUMA & SKIN CONDITIONS THAT CAUSE ULCERS

Ulcers and scabs are perhaps one of the most common reasons for anxiety concerning sexually transmitted infections. The key feature with this group of problems is ulceration. Ulceration is the breakdown of the skin or the moist 'mucus membranes' to reveal a raw, red, weeping surface underneath. Blisters and scabs are also included here because they are often part of the ulceration sequence: Blisters are early ulcers, where the skin has lifted and the raw area underneath has filled with weeping fluid but the skin has not yet come away and there is therefore a temporary fluid-filled bubble covering the future ulcer. Scabs on the other hand are the late result of ulcers, where healing is well underway and the raw area is now covered with a rough protective layer of dried blood and serum.

Whilst it is important to recognise that some major sexually transmitted diseases (STDs) can first appear with these characteristics, it is important to appreciate that not all ulcers, blisters and scabs on the genitals are STDs and many are not serious. Careful examination and appropriate tests can distinguish the different causes.

Sorting out the pieces of the puzzle; clues for the detective

Herpes is the classic sexually transmitted infection that has ulcers as one of its main features. Other STDs including early **syphilis** and the more exotic infections—**chancroid** and **donovanosis**—can also cause ulcers and 'raw spots'. Both chancroid and donovanosis are infections of tropical areas and usually need to be considered if people have been travelling or living in the tropics.

The appearances of ulcers are among the most useful clues to identifying the problem of herpes. Typical herpes begins with tingling and warmth followed by redness, then a number of small blisters appear. These become painful, red, shallow, moist ulcers 1 to 2 millimetres in diameter. These usually dry and heal after a few days.

Syphilis, on the other hand, is usually a single, larger, round, moist, painless ulcer between a half and one centimetre in diameter and lasts for a few weeks. The area under the ulcer, is usually very firm and this is described by some people as like a button hidden underneath the ulcer (if the ulcer belongs to someone else use gloves and wash hands, because the fluid coming from the ulcer contains the organism that causes syphilis and is infectious). At the ulcer stage, syphilis blood tests will be negative and diagnosis is made by examining a microscopic sample of fluid from the ulcer under a 'dark-ground' microscope (see Chapter 8).

Chancroid causes a more ragged, irregular, painful ulcer and is diagnosed by taking a sample with a cotton swab-stick and growing it in the laboratory on 'Hammond's medium'. Donovanosis, in contrast, causes moist, red, 'meaty' raised areas, and is diagnosed by examining a 'crush' preparation under the microscope stained with a special stain (Giemsa stain). Unlike a true ulcer, it is raised instead of being a hole in the skin. Herpes will be covered in more detail below. Syphilis is described in detail in Chapter 8.

Sexual activity that is unusually enthusiastic or where the skin is unusually delicate may also leave small raw, tender and weeping abrasions and may be mistaken for a sexually transmitted infection such as herpes. Sometimes the skin can become more prone to repeated tearing when stretched, such as during intercourse or masturbation, and this can be painful and worrying. A careful history and examination may be needed to establish the underlying reason for the skin being more prone to splitting or tearing. Repeated tearing can be the result of the skin being more delicate due to some skin conditions such as psoriasis or dermatitis. The doctor therefore needs to look for skin problems on other parts of the body and check for a history of dermatitis or childhood eczema. Low oestrogen levels after menopause and during breast feeding can result in similar problems. Repeated tearing can also occur because the skin is less elastic. This is sometimes the case when there is a low grade wart virus infection even though no obvious warts are present. Often the skin will split repeatedly at the same spot and this can be mistaken for herpes. Typically these repeated splits will occur at the frenulum of the penis in men (the band of skin that joins the foreskin to the underside of the penis) and in women where the labia (vaginal lips) meet in front of the vagina and between the vagina and the anus.

Allergies and irritants can cause a variety of genital skin problems and these may become raw and ulcerated. Severe allergy to some drugs, such as sulphur drugs, and to some foods can result in marked symptoms involving the entire body including the genitals. Typical symptoms of allergy include redness, swollen white patches and itching (hives) and in extreme cases blistering in the moist areas of the eyes, mouth, rectum, vagina and penis (Stevens-Johnston Syndrome). Alternately, some medications can cause local reactions known as 'fixed drug reactions'. In this case soon after taking a medication such as tetracycline or doxycycline there will be local tingling of a small, coin-sized area which in a few hours becomes red and may even become moist and raw. This affected patch, which is often but not always on the genitals, will last several days after the medication is discontinued and will usually recur at the same place whenever a similar drug is taken . Confusion sometimes occurs because the reaction can occur during treatment for a sexually transmitted infection and the individual being treated may incorrectly think that the infection is getting worse or that a new infection has occurred.

Irritants in direct contact with the genitals can also cause problems. Occasionally, an individual will complain of fluctuating, red, scaling patches on the thighs or genitals, usually persisting around the same area. The doctor should consider an allergy to the nickel studs in jeans or to the nickel in genital adornments such as studs and ring. On the other hand, a person who suspects that he or she has a sexually transmitted infection may attempt to treat him/herself by applying disinfectant! This can lead to severe burns with considerable red, raw, peeling, weeping areas of skin. A similar appearance is sometimes seen in people who have been over-enthusiastic with the paint used to treat warts. Wart paint is designed to cause a chemical 'burn'. Normal skin will also be burned by this paint and because normal skin is not as thick as wart infected skin, the burns may well be more severe. Clear instructions and considerable care needs to be taken when applying wart paint. Local allergy can also be due to sensitivity to latex or lubricants used in condoms. Genuine sensitivity is extremely unusual to condoms and so a thorough search should be made for alternative explanations before concluding that this is the problem. In the case of a genuine allergy, plastic condoms would be a reasonable alternative, but these can be difficult to obtain. Condoms derived from animal gut are not recommended as they are not thought to provide satisfactory protection against viral sexually transmitted infections.

Herpes in detail

The herpes family of viruses consists of six members of which only two are associated with genital herpes infections. These two are known as *Herpes simplex* types 1 and 2. While much effort has been put into debating the differences between type 1 and type 2 herpes, the infections due to them are much more similar than they are different.

Herpes infection can involve the mouth, the genitals, or skin and moist surfaces (mucous membranes) anywhere else on the body, and the basic pattern of infection is similar for all these sites. The virus is usually first contracted following direct contact with a herpes infection on the skin or moist surface of another person. The site where the infection occurs depends on what part of the anatomy comes into direct contact with the virus: the infection can affect the mouth and lips if an individual kisses somebody with a lip infection or has oral sex with someone with a genital infection. Conversely, the infection will affect the genitals if an individual has intercourse with someone with a genital infection or has oral sex with someone with a lip infection.

It takes on average six days from the time of coming into contact with the herpes infection to the time of developing symptoms. However, this can be as short as a day and as long as a couple of weeks. This is known as the incubation period. The first infection is usually the worst, although some people can have first infections with very minor symptoms or no symptoms at all. Typically, the infected individual becomes aware of a tender area of skin that develops small blisters (known as vesicles), which soon burst to form underlying red, tender, raw areas (herpes ulcers). The ulcers then dry and become crusted. Scabs form and within a few days the attack heals. At the time of the ulcers in first episode herpes, there may also be a fever, headache and symptoms a little like the 'flu'. At its most severe, the first episode of herpes can result in extensive, shallow, painful, red ulcers, swollen glands, fever and feeling generally unwell. In extreme cases there can be a transient meningitis with headache, neck-stiffness and discomfort on exposure to bright light (photophobia). This can be treated with the drug, acyclovir but is usually transient and will resolve spontaneously without complications. The ulcers may make eating uncomfortable if they involve the mouth and they may make passing urine difficult if they involve the vagina or penis. Occasionally, people with severe symptoms need to be admitted to hospital.

Following the first attack of herpes, the virus becomes dormant in the body. In some people it can reactivate and the sores can recur. Recurring episodes of herpes tend to occur less and less commonly and more mildly. The first attack is usually the worst and any further outbreaks tend to result in mild local sores with no generalised symptoms such as fever or headache. Reactivation occurs because at the time of the first episode, in addition to infecting the skin, the virus also infects the nerves that lie under the infected skin. Once in the nerve, the virus moves up the nerve and after the attack is over the virus can lie silently in the base of the nerve (the nerve ganglion). At a later time, the virus can be triggered into activity and move down the nerves to the skin where the original infection occurred. This will result in reactivated herpes sores. When the virus starts moving down the nerves it can stimulate a feeling of tingling, warmth or heat that seems to be coming from the skin where the nerves end (this is known as referred sensation). People who have had several herpes attacks learn to recognise these early symptoms as a sign that they are about to have another attack even before any blisters or sores appear. This sensation is known as a prodrome. What triggers the virus into activity again is poorly understood, but it is probably due both to properties of the virus and to a problem of immunity. In particular, people with poor immune systems or in a 'run-down' state of health are more likely to have repeated, prolonged or more severe attacks of herpes.

The saying that 'love is often fleeting but herpes is for life' is well known. However, this concept is a source of anxiety for some patients: Occasionally, people with first infections take this to imply that the current painful sores will persist for life! This is not the case. It is also important and reassuring for infected people to understand that it can remain permanently dormant; there are people who have no recurrences. On the other hand, in those in whom there are recurrences (60-90% in the first year), there needs to be a clear understanding that the usual pattern is that recurrences become less and less common and more and more mild over time and that the first episode is usually the worst. The exception to this rule seems to be when there is some underlying health problem or the person is 'run-down'. The logical implication of this is that if infected people maintain good health, recurrences may be reduced.

Sonia, 37, had never had a sexually transmitted infection while her girlfriend of five years, Anna, had herpes a short time before their relationship started. Anna and Sonia always took precuations against STD transmission. In particular, they used dental dams—rectangular pieces of latex rubber that fit snugly over a woman's genitals—although they knew these are not foolproof in protecting against herpes.

One morning, Sonia noticed tingling, warmth and stinging near the opening of her urethra which was more uncomfortable when she urinated. Examining herself with a mirror she saw several shallow, red, moist raw areas. Suspecting this was herpes, she decided to see her doctor before things got worse.

Her doctor agreed that Sonia appeared to have herpes and prescribed acyclovir. A sample taken from a raw area came back from the laboratory three days later with a positive test result. By that stage, the herpes had almost healed because Sonia had taken action early.

Problems can occur for the person or for a relationship if it is incorrectly assumed that a particular episode is the first ever attack. This is because the first attack requires direct contact with someone with herpes but repeat episodes don't, because they are due to reactivation of the virus that has survived silently following the first attack. An individual may mistakenly assume his or her partner has been unfaithful when in fact a long-standing herpes infection has been reactivated.

What about the difference between type 1 and type 2 herpes and mouth and genital herpes? In the past, considerable emphasis has been placed on the differences between Herpes simplex types 1 and 2. Unfortunately, over-emphasising these differences can be the source of considerable anxiety and confusion for patients and for many health workers and it is often more productive to emphasise their similarities which far outweigh any differences. The key to understanding these problems is to recognise that herpes simplex type 2 and genital herpes were unnecessarily stigmatised during the early 1970s and '80s. This had a significant influence on peoples' perceptions of herpes. In essence, people with mouth herpes may get regular attacks which are on full view and which do not cause huge problems for most people. On the other hand, people with genital herpes, which only needs to be on view if the person chooses, often feel despair and depression: It is not unusual for them to feel that genital herpes marks the end of ever having a social or sexual life and any aspirations to marry or form a relationship. This is never the response to mouth herpes which can also be passed from partner to partner during intimate contact!

The difference between types 1 and 2 herpes is most noticeable in the laboratory where they produce slightly different patterns in cell culture tests. Subtle differences in their surface structures can also be detected by tests using antibodies (serology). But even in the laboratory there are considerable similarities and many tests cannot reliably identify any difference. Type 1 herpes has been traditionally associated with mouth herpes, whereas type 2 herpes has been traditionally linked with genital herpes. However, these are interchangeable and herpes type 2 is now being increasingly seen on the mouth and type 1 increasingly seen on the genitals.

Oral (mouth) herpes is usually first contracted in childhood as a result of being kissed by someone else with herpes of the mouth. As already mentioned, the first episode is usually the worst and the child will often be irritable and unwell and have fever and lots of blisters, ulcers and sores in the mouth and around the lips. This is sometimes known as 'fever blisters' and will clear up in a few days to a couple of weeks. The virus will then be silent until the next time the child becomes ill such as when he or she has a cold. The virus may then break out in a small area on the mouth and usually does not cause symptoms such as fever or a feeling of illness. This stage is often known as 'cold sores'. These sores may recur every now and then, particularly when the child has some other health problem, but the episodes will become less common and less severe with each outbreak. Even though cold sores are common in children they are uncommon and usually quite mild in adults.

Genital herpes is a similar story except that now the time frame is later; the first infection usually occurring when the person becomes sexually active in his or her late teens and early twenties. At that time, for people who have never had oral herpes, the first episode of genital herpes is often quite severe, just as it was in the child with fever blisters. However, in people who have had prior cold sores, the first episode of genital herpes can be quite mild and may even go unnoticed or unrecognised. This is because, infection of one site with one type of herpes does produce (imperfect) immunity that reduces the severity of infection at another site with the other type. In light of this, where the 'source' partner is 'blamed', remember that he or she may well have been totally unaware of being infected or of being able to pass it on. Indeed, it is often the 'fault' of the treating doctor who has failed to diagnose past episodes having labelled them as repeated attacks of thrush!

Future outbreaks of genital herpes follow a pattern similar to childhood cold-sores, with each episode becoming less and less frequent and less severe. Typically, the infection may be troublesome in the first year or so, but then becomes infrequent and mild. For the vast majority of people with herpes, the infection is no more than nuisance value.

Diagnosis of herpes depends on recognition of the typical pattern of infection and appropriate testing for the virus. A story of a tender raw area that keeps on reappearing in approximately the same area should arouse suspicions of herpes. If the raw area is preceded by tiny blisters that become red, shallow, tender ulcers that dry and become scabs and heal in a few days, then the diagnosis of herpes would seem likely. This can be confirmed by growing the virus in cell culture. In order to culture the virus, a sample is taken by rolling a cotton swab stick in the fluid from a blister or ulcer. The swab can then be placed in cell culture, that is, when a single layer of human cells is artificially grown in a tube containing nutrients. A few days after the sample is added to the tube, characteristic damage to the cells will appear if the virus was present and has infected and attacked the cells. This test is not without its problems. The virus needs to be kept alive until it reaches the laboratory. This necessitates placing the sample into an appropriate fluid and transporting the sample from the clinic to the lab as quickly as possible. The virus also needs to be active at the time of taking the specimen. Even if the person is infected, it is most unlikely that the test will detect herpes if the sample is taken from healed herpes or normal skin. A third probem is that many laboratories do not have cell culture facilities. Alternative tests include detecting herpes by special microscopic techniques (immunofluorscence and electron microscopy) and by special assays (Elisa tests). These tests too are imperfect. Whatever test is used, remember that a positive test diagnoses herpes fairly reliably, but a negative test simply means that the virus was not detected. Any individual with suspected herpes should be advised to return immediately for further testing should the sores return.

Blood tests are also available for detection of herpes, but these currently have limited uses. This is because they give no indication as to where or when the infection occurred and do not reliably distinguish between types 1 and 2 infections. Most adults have had oral herpes, which will be detected by the tests. Perhaps the most useful feature of the test is if it gives a negative finding. In this case the person has never been infected with herpes. But, even this needs to be interpreted carefully because it can take a couple of weeks for the test to produce a positive result after an individual is infected. Therefore, if blood is taken around the time a person has his or her first attack of herpes, a second blood test should be taken in a few weeks time in order to give the test time to become positive.

On the question of precautions, the infection is spread through direct contact with infected sores: prevention aims at preventing this from happening. This can be achieved by avoiding sexual intercourse during an attack or by using condoms if the lesions can be adequately covered. Condoms are good protection against herpes providing they are used properly. However prevention can be difficult because episodes may be so mild as to go unnoticed and occasionally the virus can be passed on without any sign of an attack. For this reason, some STD workers recommend that condoms be used regardless of whether or not an attack is thought to be occurring. This also reduces the chance of contracting other infections. Whether herpes can also be spread through contact with contaminated objects is unlikely. The herpes virus is enclosed in a fragile envelope which is essential if it is to cause infections. This envelope also makes the virus very susceptible to rapid inactivation once it has left the security of the body. For the virus to spread via inanimate objects it probably needs to be present in large amounts, fresh and moist, and to come into contact with broken skin. This theoretical risk does cause anxiety for some individuals and it is not unreasonable for them to wash hands and objects that come into contact with lesions.

There are basically four key elements to the treatment of herpes. The first is prevention of infection. Second, because the state of an individual's health seems so important to the activity of herpes the next approach is directed at reducing stress, improving nutrition, treating underlying health problems and taking general measures to improve health. Many people at this point get great comfort from joining a herpes self-help group. Third, local treatment with betadine skin antiseptic is useful to dry ulcers, promote healing and stop bacteria from aggravating the lesions. As well, xylocaine jelly or xylocaine ointment or pain-killing medications may help. Fourth, suppression of herpes with antiviral drugs such as acyclovir may prove valuable. This is a useful drug that has only rarely been associated with side-effects. Acyclovir has been shown to speed healing, prevent new sores from developing, reduce the duration of symptoms and reduce the amount of virus produced during the infection. Unfortunately, acyclovir is only a suppressive drug and does not cure the infection: an individual can redevelop herpes after the acyclovir course has been completed. Thus when using acyclovir, it is important to try to improve general health in the hope that this will lessen the chance of a relapse. Acyclovir has been suggested as a possible treatment for herpes when taken long-term. Unfortunately, however, the drug is far too expensive for the average person to contemplate prolonged administration; its ability to suppress the virus is not perfect; there is a theoretical risk of encouraging the development of viruses resistant to acyclovir thus rendering it useless for future treatment; and many STD workers feel uncomfortable recommending prolonged treatment with a relatively new drug. In addition most episodes of herpes are so mild that using acyclovir is not necessary. Currently, therefore, it is thought best to reserve acyclovir for people with the very severe first episodes of herpes, for those with frequent recurrences (ie more than ten per year) and for people with suppressed immunity.

Herpes is a special problem for people with very poor or undeveloped immune systems. This includes the newborn, people with HIV/AIDS and people who are taking immune suppressing drugs following organ transplantation. In the case of people with AIDS and people who have had transplants, herpes can cause prolonged severe infection known as 'chronic mucocutaneous herpes'. Fortunately this can be fairly easily controlled by taking continual acyclovir tablets. In the case of the newborn, the virus can be contracted during childbirth if the mother has active genital infection. Under these circumstances, the child will have little resistance to the virus, which can cause a serious, life-threatening infection if left untreated. It is therefore important for mothers who have had herpes to tell the doctor responsible for the childbirth of this. The doctor can then test for the virus and take precautions if it is active at the time of labour. Precautions against herpes-spread during childbirth include masking any obvious herpes or delivering the baby by Caesarian section if the sores cannot be masked. Unfortunately prevention is made more difficult because most babies with herpes are born to mothers who did not know they were infected. Health workers therefore need to be alert to this possibility so they can make an early diagnosis at the first sign of problems in a baby. If diagnosed early, the infection can be suppressed and the problems for the child minimised with intravenous acyclovir treatment.

Chancroid, donovanosis and LGV

These infections are uncommon in Western countries and are most often seen in the third world and the tropics although outbreaks can occur in any country including northern Australia. Often they can be distinguished by their typical appearance but occasionally they can be confused with the ulcers of herpes and syphilis. For this reason, testing for herpes and syphilis is often carried out when considering the diagnosis.

Chancroid is caused by a bacterium called *Haemophilus ducreyi*. It is more common in uncircumcised men than in those who have been circumcised. The incubation period varies from one day to several weeks (average five to seven days). Sores typically begin with a tender, red warty lump that produces pus and then forms an ulcer. These ulcers are usually single but can be multiple and are usually painful, irregular and differ from herpes because they are generally deeper and larger. The groin lymph nodes are usually swollen and tender. If infection is prolonged, these nodes can develop into abscesses. Diagnosis can be confirmed by taking material from the base of the ulcer or the lymph node and gram staining it and culturing it on 'Hammond's' medium. Treatment with erythromycin tablets or ceftriaxone injection is effective.

Donovanosis is caused by a bacterium *Calymmatobacterium* *granulomatis.* The incubation period is between eight and eighty days. Sores typically begin as firm nodules, the surface of which erode to form 'beefy', raised, raw, painless areas known as granulomas. These differ from other ulcers because they are raised above the skin rather than forming a crater. If untreated, granulomas gradually enlarge and spread. Diagnosis is confirmed by taking a small sample of the granuloma and compressing it onto a glass slide. This is known as a 'crush' preparation. The slide is stained with either Giemsa or Wright stain and examined under a microscope. Alternatively, a Pap test from the area can be performed. Treatment with either tetracycline, ampicillin or cotrimoxazole is effective.

LGV is an abbreviation for **Lymphogranuloma Venereum.** LGV is an infection caused by a particular type of chlamydia called *Chlamydia trachomatis LGV strain.* This strain is unusual in Western countries and behaves differently from the chlamydia strains discussed in Chapter 4. The incubation period is between three days to three weeks. After this incubation period, a small painless sore appears at the site where the genitals became infected. This takes the form of a small fluid filled bubble, a firm nodule or an ulcer which quickly heals. After the infection seems to have healed it again reappears causing painful, swollen lymph nodes. If untreated, these nodes increase in size and form abscesses which eventually release pus through the skin. In order to make a diagnosis, the STD worker relies on the appearance of the lesion, a sample of the pus for the LGV strain of chlamydia, and testing of blood for antibodies against LGV. Treatment with doxycycline or erythromycin has proved helpful.

Chapter Seven

RED AND ITCHY AREAS: SCABIES, CRABS, TINEA, THRUSH AND OTHER SKIN CONDITIONS THAT CAUSE RASH

Historically, dermatology (the science of skin diseases) has been linked closely with venereology (the science of sexually transmitted diseases). Indeed, in the past, venereology and dermatology were part of the same discipline and this is still the case in many parts of the world. A reason for this link may be that one of the many manifestations of syphilis is a rash, and other sexually transmitted problems can also cause certain types of rash. It is common for people with rashes and itches to attend a STD specialist first to check whether or not they have a sexually-acquired infection. Perhaps this is because some rashes are viewed as a sign of sexually transmitted infections, they can trigger an attack of 'the guilts' or because people want the possibility of an embarrasing sexually transmitted infection excluded before seeing their regular doctor.

Some sexually transmitted infections can cause rashes as part of their pattern of infection. Infestations such as pubic lice and scabies can cause an itchy rash throughout areas where there is pubic hair. Tinea and thrush can cause red, itchy patches in moist areas of the skin such as in skin folds between toes, under breasts, in the groin, under the foreskin, in the vagina and around the vaginal lips (labia). Skin conditions such as dermatitis and psoriasis can affect the skin of the genitals as well as elsewhere and sometimes, they can affect the genitals alone without involving the rest of the body. Because the skin of the genitals is more delicate, often more darkly pigmented and rarely exposed to sunshine, the appearance of such skin conditions may differ according to which part of the body is affected. Confusion also arises when the problem is seen around the genitals for the first time even though other parts of the body may have been affected for some time previously. To add to the confusion, the first sign of a problem may appear following some sort of irritation to the genitals. The irritation may have been very mild and may even follow sexual intercourse particularly when mild abrasions have affected the genital skin. Minor trauma is a well known trigger for the appearance of skin conditions at a previously unaffected site. This is known as the 'Koebner' phenomenon.

The appearance of red and itchy areas involving the genitals often leads to fear of a sexually transmitted infection. Usually a careful history and examination by an experienced venereologist can clarify the problem. Some of the tools used to unravel the puzzle include taking a careful history of past skin problems, any new drugs and medications that are being taken, food allergies, previous skin complaints and sexual activities. The examination may reveal skin changes similar to those on other parts of the body or changes that are characteristic of conditions when they involve the genitals. Where there is any doubt and the condition appears important enough to warrant further investigation, additional tests may be carried out. Tests that should be considered include taking a cotton swab of any ulcer to test for herpes; bacterial, candida and fungal culture; blood tests for syphilis; and occasionally a small biopsy with local anaesthetic so that the affected skin can be examined under the microscope.

Whilst the AIDS virus, HIV, can occasionally cause specific rashes, jumping to conclusions should be avoided. A detailed discussion of HIV can be found in Chapter 8.

Scabies and lice

Technically, problems due to these tiny animals are called infestations rather than infections because they are due to mites and insects rather than microorganisms such as bacteria and viruses. Both of the culprits are only around one mm across and are best viewed under a microscope. The cause of scabies can then clearly be identified as an eight legged mite (called *Sarcoptes scabei*) and the cause of pubic lice can be seen to be the pubic louse, a six legged insect (called *Pthirus pubis*). Head lice are more common in children whereas pubic lice are more common in sexually active young adults. Head lice are due to *Pediculus humanus* and are microscopically and clinically different from pubic lice.

The difference between **scabies** and **lice** is important and provides the clue to diagnosis. Pubic lice live on the surface of the skin and

One day at work, Tony found that he could not stop an itch beneath his underpants. During his tea break, he went to the toilet and found a number of itchy red 'pimples' in his pubic hair and two itchy red spots on the head of his penis.

Tony recognised the problem as scabies from a previous experience. Once before he had similar symptoms and spent ages trying to work out the problem. Everything became clear when he was told that the mites involved burrow under the skin, thereby causing the itch.

Tony also knew that a treatment for scabies does not need a doctor's prescription, but he decided to go to the STD clinic for a check anyway just in case there were any other problems.

anchor themselves firmly to the base of hairs where they can be seen as tiny fawn-brown blemishes or scales about a millimetre across. Careful examination reveals that these scales are tiny lice that cling firmly to the base of hairs and crawl across the skin when dislodged. They can be found wherever there is pubic hair and lay eggs which adhere firmly to the shaft of hairs. These eggs, known as 'nits', are often the first clue to infestation with lice. The eggs usually look a whitish colour on dark hair and a brownish colour on light hair and to the untrained eye, may initially be mistaken for dandruff (seborrhoeic dermatitis). Unlike dandruff, the lice are attached firmly to the hair and are difficult to dislodge. The main symptom of pubic lice is a mild to moderate itchy rash. Closer examination reveals that the rash consists mainly of scratch marks.

The mites responsible for scabies, on the other hand, live in shallow burrows under the skin where they lay their eggs. This causes scabies to be itchier than a pubic lice infestation and more difficult to find. Also, in addition to the scratch marks, scabies usually produces a rash wherever there are burrows. In a typical case, the rash consists of red raised spots (papules) around three to four mm in diameter around the pubic region. These red spots are due to a skin reaction at the site of the burrow. The burrows, and hence the rash, may also be found between the buttocks, on the forearms and even between the finger webs. In men the scabies rash often appears on the glans (head) of the penis. Because scabies burrow under the skin, the mite cannot usually be seen unless a burrow is identified and opened up with a sterile pin. Burrows can be seen better by putting some indian ink on the skin. The ink will leak into the burrow and leave a dark line for up to one cm along the burrow. This can be seen through the skin after the ink on the surface is wiped off.

Both scabies and lice are passed from person to person by intimate skin to skin contact. They are unlikely to be passed by other means. However, it is usual to recommend that bedclothes and underwear be changed and washed at the time of treatment. This is to ensure that the treatment is successful and that the person doesn't become reinfested. It also implies that the infestation can be passed on by shared underwear and bed clothes.

Treatment is with gamma benzene hexachloride or benzyl benzoate cream or lotion. These are essentially insecticides in a moistursing cream and should be applied to the affected area from the neck down and left overnight and removed the next morning in the shower or bath. In the case of lice, combing the hair after treatment will also assist in removing nits. Treatment should be repeated after seven to ten days to remove any developing nits that were not cleared by the first treatment.

The preparations mentioned above are nontoxic if used according to the instructions and usually do not require a prescription. However, a medical checkup is recommended in order to confirm the diagnosis and to check for other infections. The treatments should not be used on children under two years of age, or above the neck, and should not be applied more than twice in the space of a week. If the infestation reappears, a check should be made for a source such as an untreated partner or unchanged underwear or bedclothes. In the case of scabies, itching will persist for up to two weeks because it takes some time for the skin to shed and the burrows to disappear. Itching for up to two weeks after scabies has been treated does not imply that the treatment has failed.

Tinea and thrush skin infections

Tinea and **thrush (candida** or **monilia)** are related infections because both belong to the 'fungus' family and both share some characteristics when they infect skin. Both can cause infections in skin folds wherever there is warm, moist skin particularly where the moisture and rubbing have caused mild skin damage (maceration) and particularly in hot climates or where tight or heavy clothing causes over-heating and sweating. The most likely skin folds to be affected by tinea are between the toes where it is known as athletes foot (**tinea pedis**) and in the groin (**tinea cruris**). Thrush and tinea can also affect other sites such as under the breasts and between skin folds particularly in people who are overweight, and under the foreskin in men who are not circumcised.

Tinea is not a sexually transmitted infection but often comes to the notice of the STD specialist when it involves the groin. The infection is spread by coming into contact with one of the several microscopic fungi that cause tinea (*Trichophyton, Microsporum* or *Epidermophyton*). Classically, the first contact with tinea is on the floor of shared showers where the fungus survives in the warm moist conditions and can spread from the feet of one person to the feet of another.

On the toes, the typical pattern of tinea symptoms is of itching and scaling between the third and fourth toes (the big toe is the first toe). The symptoms usually occur in cycles and sometimes there will be no itch and very little scaling. A few weeks later, itching may be intense with peeling and even weeping fluid from between the affected toes. Tinea can spread from the toes to the groin probably on fingers that have scratched infected toes. The groin is a 'safe haven' for the tinea where it can lodge between the skin folds gaining a foothold because the skin has been softened by sweating and abraded by the edges of moist underwear. In the groin it produces a rash several centimetres in diameter, most often in men in the fold between the scrotum and the top of the thigh. Depending on the activity of the tinea, the rash varies between a very fine scaling that is almost unnoticeable, to a dry, scaling red zone with a clear border between normal and infected skin, to an itchy, red, weeping infection. Usually, this is as far as the infection progresses but occasionally, the tinea can be spread to other skin folds, the hair and nails. Sometimes it can form a very resistant infection in the hair or beard where it is often known as '**ringworm**'. Ringworm is an unfortunate name because it has nothing to do with worms.

The diagnosis of tinea is usually clear from the appearance of the rash, but if there is any doubt it can be confirmed by collecting a sample of the scales or scrapings from affected skin or nail and hair clippings, examining them microscopically, and culturing them for fungi. It is important that the samples from affected sites, such as the active margin of a rash and the damaged portion of hair and nails are collected in a sterile container—otherwise the fungus may not be detected.

The treatment of tinea and candida is essentially the same, both being fungi. Antifungal creams such as clotrimazole or miconazole or nystatin can be applied to the affected skin twice a day. Only apply enough to cover the infection as excessive cream seems to keep the area moist and healing may not be as rapid. In addition to treatment with antifungal creams, attention should be directed towards correcting the reason for the infection flaring up in the first place. The infections almost always occur because organisms find themselves in a warm moist environment in which they can grow. Furthermore, whilst these infections can occur in people with good health, the organism is aided if the person's immune defences are down. Natural defences to these infections include dry skin which can be damaged by being continually damp, other organisms on the skin which can prevent the tinea from becoming established (and which can be adversely affected by antibiotics) and a poor immune system. Preventive measures should therefore be directed to altering these predisposing factors. Keeping affected areas dry will reduce the chance of relapse after the course of antifungal cream is completed. Regularly changing underwear; wearing airy, loose, non-synthetic clothing to reduce sweating; careful drying after showering, swimming, using the toilet and strenuous physical activity; and losing weight if obesity is a problem, will all aid treatment and reduce the chance of relapse. (Some people find that a hairdryer is also very useful). Underlying medical problems may have played a role also; diabetes, and treatment with antibiotics may have triggered the infection. This is one of many good arguments for avoiding antibiotics when they are unnecesssary—but it is not an argument for not using antibiotics when treatment is important.

For tinea infections of hair or nails that resist treatment, griseofulvin tablets should be considered. Griseofulvin is deposited in the skin, hair and nails where it acts against the fungus. It will not work against candida. Because it takes months for the old hair and nails to be replaced with new growth that contains the drug, the medication needs to be administered for many months and occasionally has side-effects. For intractable candida, oral tablets such as ketoconazole and fluconazole are sometimes effective.

Related problems that can cause confusion

Tinea versicolor and **erythrasma** are sometimes confused with tinea.

Tinea versicolor is a fungal infection with a very different appearance from tinea. The usual pattern is of oval areas a centimetre or so in diameter with loss of pigmentation in people who are tanned or who have dark skin and slightly darkened patches of skin in people who have very light skin. The patches occur most commonly across the shoulders and upper arms. The patches are usually dry and have a very fine scaling that may be difficult to detect but can be best demonstrated by gentle scratching. Usually the patches have no symptoms: they are not itchy and do not become inflamed. An effective treatment involves using Selenium sulphide (Selsun) shampoo. The infection will also respond to clotrimazole cream.

Erythrasma, on the other hand, looks similar to typical tinea but, unlike tinea, is due to bacteria (*Corynebacterium minutissimum*). It therefore requires different treatment. Erythrasma affects similar areas to tinea: the groin and between the toes. The patches are usually irregular, clearly delineated from surrounding skin, red to red-brown and dry with mild scaling. If there is any doubt, the STD specialist will take scrapings for fungal culture to check for tinea and will have the patches examined under a 'wood's lamp', if this is available. A wood's lamp is a special form of ultraviolet lamp that causes erythrasma to glow pink-red whereas tinea usually does not glow or on occasion glows green. Erythrasma is treated effectively with erythromycin tablets.

Other skin conditions: Dermatitis, Psoriasis and Drug Reactions

Dermatitis and **psoriasis** are not sexually transmitted infections, but that does not stop them from sometimes affecting the genitals and being mistaken for STDs. Both can produce red, scaling rashes and dermatitis can often weep.

Dermatitis can be the skin's response to certain irritating substances and it only occurs in susceptible people. In others, the substance is harmless and causes no response at all. The exposure can be by direct contact with the skin of the genitals or by indirect contact such as by eating certain foods. This can then give rise to a rash that can affect the genitals and other parts of the body. The range of substances that can trigger such reactions is extensive and includes foods, drugs, chemicals, cosmetics, toiletries and plants. Even the nickel in the studs in denim trousers or genital jewellery can produce a local reaction in some people!

Condoms and associated lubricants are very uncommon causes of irritation and caution is recommended before concluding that the dermatitis is due to condom allergy. Irritation may simply be mechanical and may respond to a change in the technique of using the condom or lubricant or to a change in the brand of the lubricant. Changing from latex condoms to 'natural' condoms made from animal intestine is not usually recommended. Animal intestine condoms have been shown to contain pores large enough to allow the passage of viruses. Newer plastic condoms may be an alternative but are currently only available from specialised stores such as sex shops.

Careful detective work is required in order to track down the substance that has triggered the problem. Avoiding contact with the substance then overcomes the problem. Sometimes no agent can be found and the dermatitis is then said to be 'endogenous'. Avoiding substances that worsen the irritation, applying soothing creams to dry areas or applying drying preparations to moist areas are usually recommended. Sometimes corticosteroid creams that have the effect of suppressing the inflammation may be tried. Caution needs to be exercised when using these creams because whilst they are effective for treating dermatitis, they will make infections like herpes worse. If a skin problem worsens with steroid creams, a problem other than dermatitis, probably involving an infection, should be considered.

Certain medications can produce unexpected reactions in some susceptible people. Allergic reactions can result in a variety of rashes. Sometimes the reaction can cause a widespread rash that is itchy, or large itchy white raised areas called hives may occur. Some substances can 'sensitise' the skin and only cause a rash after the skin is exposed to the sun. This is called a photosensitivity reaction. Rarely, these allergic reactions can be severe and life threatening (anaphylaxis and Stevens-Johnson Syndrome) but usually they are mild and mainly of nuisance value.

Perhaps the most common drug reaction seen at an STD clinic is a 'fixed-drug reaction'. This usually follows a course of tetracycline or doxycycline—the usual antibiotics prescribed for chlamydia. The reaction typically starts within a couple of hours of taking the medication, commencing with tingling and itching that is localised to a patch of skin the size of a coin. The area soon becomes red and irritated and may even blister and become raw. The reaction remains confined to that one site and persists for around two weeks after ceasing use of the drug. Recommencing the drug causes the patch to reappear at the same place. The reaction can occur anywhere but often involves the genitals. The reaction can be very disconcerting for the patient who may have been taking tetracycline for an STD. It can be confused with infections such as herpes and sometimes an individual concludes that the treatment is not adequate or the 'VD' is getting worse or is incurable.

The treatment of a fixed drug reaction is to stop using antibiotics and attend the prescribing doctor for confirmation of the diagnosis. Rather than ceasing treatment altogether, it is important to change and replace the antibiotic with another medication such as erythromycin. If the cause of the problem does not seem to be an antibiotic, any medication or new substance taken recently, including 'alternative' medicine preparations, should be stopped and the response noted.

Chapter Eight

SEXUALLY TRANSMITTED INFECTIONS THAT TRAVEL IN THE BLOODSTREAM: HEPATITIS, SYPHILIS, AIDS AND OTHERS

Despite being transmitted during intercourse, some sexually transmitted diseases (STDs) can cause serious infections elsewhere in the body with minor or no involvement of the sexual organs. The most important of these are hepatitis, AIDS and syphilis. While each of these infections are very different, they share some characteristics which influence their disease pattern: for each, infection involving the genitals is not a prominent feature; each can have a long period when infection is silent; each can be passed on during this time of silence; and for each the diagnosis is best confirmed through blood testing.

Hepatitis

Hepatitis is inflammation of the liver, an organ situated in the upper abdomen, tucked behind the lower ribs and below the diaphragm. It carries out vital metabolic functions; destroying, manufacturing and converting substances in the circulation into harmless or useful by-products. Inflammation of the liver interferes with these processes, and the by-products of day-to-day living accumulate in the blood. The affected individual feels unwell and the by-products of degenerating red blood cells (called bilirubin) accumulate and cause a yellowish discoloration of the skin and moist surfaces. This is known as jaundice. Jaundice is most noticeable in the whites of the eyes (sclera) where the green-yellow colouration is known as icterus. When the liver is inflamed, it can swell and become uncomfortable. Its enlargement can be felt as a firmness in the abdomen below the ribs.

Hepatitis can have a number of causes, many of which are not sexually transmitted. For example, a number of drugs and chemicals can cause inflammation of the liver, in which case the hepatitis is due to poisoning or to allergic reactions rather than to an infection. On the other hand, a number of viruses can cause infectious hepatitis. These include the *hepatitis A, B, C, D* and *E* viruses. In addition, some viruses that normally do not produce obvious hepatitis can cause the infection in some people. These viruses include the glandular fever virus (also known as the *Epstein Barr Virus* or *EBV*) and the *cytomegalovirus (or CMV)*.

Although **hepatitis A** is caused by a viral infection, it is usually not spread sexually. The hepatitis A virus is an intestinal infection and spreads by the 'faecal-oral' route. That is, it is passed in the faeces and, in the presence of poor hygiene, it can contaminate water, food and utensils and if swallowed can infect the next person. While not normally a sexually transmitted infection, hepatitis A can occasionally be passed through practices such as oral sex. This depends, of course, on one person already being infected. Prevention depends on good hygiene such as hand washing and on avoiding handling food. Hepatitis A can also be prevented by giving immunoglobulin injections either before a potential exposure or immediately after an exposure. (Immmunoglobulins are antibodies extracted from the blood of people who are immune to a particular type of infectious agent.) In the case of Hepatitis A exposure, this approach is of limited use. A new hepatitis vaccine is now available.

Hepatitis E is a newly discovered virus that spreads in a similar manner to hepatitis A, while **hepatitis B, C and D** share a number of characteristics.

Hepatitis B is caused by a virus that can be passed on during sexual contact, by injection of infected blood, and from mother to child during childbirth. In this respect, hepatitis B is passed on in a similar manner to human immune deficiency virus—HIV (the AIDS virus). However, hepatitis B is easier to transmit than HIV, and can even occasionally be passed in saliva. Following infection, there is a 'silent' or incubation period that lasts for a few weeks to a few months before the symptoms of hepatitis appear, sometimes preceded by joint aches and pains. This is known as a 'prodrome.' The typical symptoms of hepatitis include nausea, pale bowel motions, feeling generally unwell, dark urine and jaundice. The dark urine and pale faeces can be explained by the accumulation in the blood of the by-product of the breakdown of red blood cells (bilirubin). This is normally filtered by the liver into the intestine thus causing the brown colour of the faeces. However, when the liver is not functioning properly because of hepatitis, the bilirubin accumulates in the blood and causes jaundice. When the jaundice reaches a certain level, the bilirubin is lost through the kidneys where it causes darkening of the urine. Because the bile is no longer being lost into the faeces, the bowel motions become pale.

About 95% of adults who contract hepatitis B overcome the infection and develop permanent immunity. Unfortunately, the other 5% are unable to do so and remain permanently infected. These people are known as hepatitis B carriers. In some of these individuals, the virus remains relatively dormant and causes no great problems; in others the virus may have a low activity and cause chronic

---

Paul and his girlfriend, Karen, had always used condoms during sex. Twelve years earlier, Karen had used injectable drugs. She was never addicted but used 'speed' (injectable amphetamines) on a couple of occasions at parties.

In those days, no-one had heard of AIDS and no-one she knew had ever had hepatitis. In fact, everyone seemed healthy and needles were commonly shared.

Six months after Paul and Karen started having sex, Paul felt unwell. First, his joints ached for a few days. Then he felt nauseated and lost his appetite. He also noticed his urine was very dark. Then, the whites of his eyes became yellow, and his skin took on the same tinge.

The local doctor diagnosed hepatitis and took a sample of blood. He also suggested that Karen should have some blood taken and advised her to start a course of vaccination against hepatitis.

Two days later, the preliminary blood test results came through, which showed that Paul had acute hepatitis B and Karen was also infected. The pattern of her blood test result suggested she had been infected for a long time and may have been carrying hepatitis B without symptoms since sharing needles years before.

The counsellor explained that hepatitis B can be passed in saliva during kissing and that partners of people who carry hepatitis B can be protected by vaccination, if they take action early enough.

hepatitis. After many years of chronic hepatitis, infected individuals may have severe scarring of the liver (cirrhosis) and even cancer of the liver (hepatoma). It should be remembered that this is an uncommon outcome of adult hepatitis B and usually only follows many years of infection.

Babies can be exposed to hepatitis at birth if their mothers have been previously infected. However if a mother has had hepatitis in the past and blood tests confirm that the infection has been completely eradicated, then there is no risk. Unlike adults, babies who are exposed to the virus have a much greater chance of developing a (mild) infection but also have a much greater chance of then becoming permanent carriers. People who become infected with hepatitis B as babies are more likely to develop complications later in life because the virus has longer to cause liver damage. Some populations start with a high rate of hepatitis B virus among mothers; there is thus a greater chance of passing it to children during birth. These children then have a greater chance of passing the virus to the next generation. Examples of populations with above-average numbers of hepatitis B carriers include some groups from South East Asia and some Mediterranean countries, as well as Aboriginal Australians.

Babies born to mothers who carry the hepatitis B virus can be protected from the infection by vaccination. It has been shown that this prevents the long term complications of carrying hepatitis B. It is therefore important that pregnant women are checked for hepatitis B infection before they give birth. If a woman is found to be infected during pregnancy, the baby should be given antibodies against hepatitis B (called hepatitis B immunoglobulin) and a course of the hepatitis B vaccine. The baby should receive the immunoglobulin as soon as possible after birth and certainly within 72 hours. The vaccine should be commenced in the first week of life and further booster doses given after one month and six months.

Similar procedures can also be followed for adults who are accidentally exposed to hepatitis B. For example, a health worker accidentally injured by a needle that has previously pierced the skin of someone with hepatitis B should be given the immunoglobulin and vaccine if he or she has not been vaccinated against hepatitis B. People who are likely to be at high risk of hepatitis B infection should consider being vaccinated routinely to avoid this situation. This includes health workers, sex workers, gay men, intra-venous drug users and people from populations with a higher-than-average rate of hepatitis B such as people from South-East Asia and Mediterranean countries, and indigenous Australians. Reduced exposure to hepatitis B infection can be achieved if individuals routinely adopt practices to do with safe sex, safe needle use and safe handling of sharp implements in health settings. Because hepatitis B can occasionally be passed in saliva, safe sex is probably not as effective against hepatitis B as it is against HIV/AIDS. For this reason, people with frequent partners and partners of people carrying hepatitis B should consider being vaccinated.

Treatment of chronic carriage of hepatitis B is currently not possible although some new approaches seem promising. These treatments are experimental but in the next few years a combination of treatments, possibly including corticosteroids and interferon, may assist in eradicating the virus. In the meantime, taking care of health and avoiding practices that damage the liver (such as heavy drinking) are thought to be important. It is also reasonable for chronic carriers to have liver function tests every now and then. If the tests are fairly normal, yearly tests are probably sufficient. If the tests are not normal more frequent testing is useful.

Hepatitis C has only recently been discovered although its existence has been suspected for some time and is now thought to be the major cause of what was previously known as non-A non-B hepatitis. There are a number of similarities between hepatitis B and hepatitis C. The hepatitis C virus is passed from person to person in much the same way as hepatitis B but seems to cause a milder hepatitis than hepatitis B. It tends to go unnoticed but is also more likely to persist in the liver for prolonged periods and, in some cases, for life (possibly up to 50% of cases). This can produce mild liver damage and, if carried for many years, hepatitis C may also lead to cirrhosis and possibly cancer of the liver. Tests for hepatitis C are new and cannot yet accurately differentiate chronic infection from past infection. The drug, interferon, may help some patienes. Checking liver function every six months or so, looking after one's health and safe sex and safe needle use are as important as they are for chronic hepatitis B.

In contrast, the **hepatitis D** virus is an unusual virus because it cannot survive without hepatitis B. Therefore, hepatitis D infections only ever occur when somebody has hepatitis B. This can occur in addition to a new hepatitis B infection or on top of pre-existing chronic hepatitis B. If the hepatitis B infection resolves then the hepatitis D infection will also resolve. This explains the two main patterns of hepatitis D infection. The first is associated with acute hepatitis B and this simply causes a more severe hepatitis that gets better as soon as the hepatitis B resolves. The second pattern is seen in a person who already has chronic hepatitis B. In this case, the hepatitis is milder but usually lasts for as long as the infection with hepatitis B, which could be for life. Long-term carriage of hepatitis D can occur in conjunction with long-term carriage of hepatitis B. The chances of developing complications in this situation are probably higher than if either type of hepatitis occurs on its own. Once again, maintaining health, avoiding substances that can damage the liver and taking precautions to avoid passing on the viruses are all important.

Hepatitis tests

The numerous tests available for hepatitis frequently cause confusion and a review of basic information about tests may help.

As with other blood tests, tests for hepatitis are divided into antibody and antigen tests. Antibodies are produced by the immune system and therefore tests for antibodies are tests for an immune response to a particular infection. The main problem with antibody tests is that the immune reaction is not immediate and while most antibody tests return a positive result within a few weeks of contact with an infectious agent, in some people, this can take up to three months. Therefore, as a general rule the 'all clear' for infections that rely on antibody tests for diagnosis cannot be given until three months has passed following contact with the infection.

Antibody tests are designed to detect either of two main types of antibody in blood: total antibody or IgM (Immunoglobulin M) antibody. IgM develops early in an infection and lasts for a few weeks and then usually disappears. Testing for IgM against a particular infection is therefore useful to detect a new infection and tells you that the exposure was recent. The second type of antibody is IgG (Immunoglobulin G) and this is the main component detected in 'total' antibody tests. This develops after IgM has appeared. Once IgG is positive it usually lasts for life, even if the infection has cleared. Total antibody tests give an indication of exposure but no indication of how recently this occurred: a positive

IgG test simply indicates exposure at some time in the past.

An antigen test detects a component of the virus causing the infection. The key components of the hepatitis B virus are its core and substances on its surface called surface antigens. Tests to detect these components are available. An antigen test usually becomes positive earlier than an antibody test because it tests for the presence of the virus rather than the body's response to the infection.

Choosing between antibody and antigen tests and between IgG and IgM tests can be difficult for health workers. But the choice is important if a person's status is to be evaluated correctly. Hepatitis B tests can be best understood by posing three important questions. The first is: Has the person ever been exposed? The best test to answer this question is the 'hepatitis B core antibody' test. This gives a positive result just before or at the time that a person develops the symptoms of hepatitis and will stay positive during the illness, during recovery and for life. It will only be negative during the incubation period; the time from when the person becomes infected to when he or she becomes ill.

If the core antibody test is positive and therefore confirms that the person has been exposed, the next question is: When did this exposure occur? This can be answered by doing the 'hepatitis B core IgM' test. If that test is positive, the infection is recent—some time over the last few months. If core IgM is negative, the infection occurred some time ago. In either case, the final question is: Has the infection been eradicated? The 'hepatitis B surface antigen' test is most capable of answering this question. If the hepatitis B surface antigen test is positive, then the virus is still present in the liver. If a positive result is obtained for six or more months, then the person is a chronic carrier. This can also be deduced by looking at the core IgM test. If the virus is present (surface antigen positive) but the core IgM is negative then it is reasonable to conclude that the person has been carrying the virus for some time.

Hepatitis C testing is less complicated but also less helpful. Currently, the only test routinely available is a test for antibodies to hepatitis C. As mentioned, the test is not capable of reliably differentiating between current and past infection and it is also not possible to conclusively distinguish between people who are carriers of the hepatitis C virus and those who have completely eradicated the infection. Therefore, at the time of writing, anybody with a positive test for hepatitis C antibodies is assumed to be infected and is asked not to donate blood. Sometimes a better idea of whether or not the person is infected can be obtained from liver function tests. These tests give an indication of how well the liver is performing. People who are carrying the hepatitis C virus may have slightly abnormal liver function tests.

Because the hepatitis D virus is dependent on the hepatitis B virus, there is no point testing for hepatitis D unless the test for hepatitis B surface antigen is first found to be positive. Tests to detect antibodies to hepatitis D may then be useful. In an acute infection antibody levels may be low and may not be detected by the test. In chronic infection, antibody levels are usually quite high.

Syphilis

Syphilis is now uncommon in many Western communities but it has not disappeared. In some parts of the United States, it has undergone a resurgence in recent years. In many non-Western countries, syphilis is still as common as it always has been. In Australia, pockets of syphilis still exist, particularly in the north of the continent and syphilis occurs sporadically elsewhere. The bacterium that causes syphilis is called *Treponaema pallidum* and is also known as a spirochaete because of its peculiar spiral shape when seen under the microscope. Spirochaetes are unusually small bacteria and, because of this, they cannot be seen using standard microscope techniques but require a 'dark ground' microscope.

Unlike hepatitis and HIV, syphilis is a bacterial infection and therefore can be treated with antibiotics (penicillin). If untreated, syphilis can persist for many years and can lead to serious complications. The complications of syphilis can be best understood by arbitrarily dividing syphilis into several stages.

Primary syphilis is the initial stage that occurs immediately following infection. Infection occurs by direct contact with infected body secretions. To be transmitted, syphilis probably needs to come into contact with broken skin or moist membranes. However, such breaks may be microscopic and, as with HIV and hepatitis B, protection from infection cannot be assumed just because obvious abrasions are not visible. The first sign of infection appears ten days to three months following infection. At this stage, a raw area or ulcer develops. This is called a chancre and is the most typical sign of the first or primary stage of syphilis. A number of characteristics of chancre can help to distinguish it from ulcers. The chancre is usually painless and single, and sits on a firm base. When fully developed, the ulcer is up to one cm in diameter and has a raised edge that forms a ridge around the ulcer. Because of the firm base, the ulcer can be picked up between the fingers as if there was a button underneath. The surface of the ulcer is raw and moist even though the chancre is usually painless. The fluid that comes from the raw surface contains numerous syphilis organisms. Therefore it is important to wear latex gloves if the chancre is to be touched. At this stage of ulcer development, syphilis blood tests are usually still negative. A diagnosis is usually confirmed by looking for spirochaetes in fluid leaking from the ulcer using 'dark-ground microscopy'.

Because the ulcer is painless and can occur in a variety of places (often hidden in the vagina or rectum), the chancre may go unreported or unnoticed. Diagnosis of the problem may then be delayed because the chancre will heal over the next few weeks.

The next phase of syphilis after the chancre heals is known as secondary syphilis. This stage is the result of generalised infection and has a variety of manifestations. Secondary syphilis typically appears as generalised symptoms such as fever, tiredness, swollen glands (lymphadenopathy), rashes and problems of the moist surfaces (mucus membranes). The symptoms of syphilis, are notoriously variable and syphilis has come to be known as the 'great mimicker' because it can be mistaken for so many other diseases. Rashes can be flat or raised, red or tan, scaling or smooth and affect almost any part of the body. The rash of secondary syphilis is well known for affecting the palms of the hands and the soles of the feet. Many other rashes avoid these sites and it was once thought that only syphilis affected the palms and soles. Whilst this is a useful sign, this is now known not to be absolute.

Secondary syphilis can also affect the mucus membranes. On these moist surfaces, syphilis can produce tiny ulcers that seem to wander across the membrane and are thus called 'snailtrack' ulcers. On the other hand, rather than producing erosions of the membrane, secondary syphilis can also produce wart-like lesions known as 'condylomata acuminata'. These occur in areas where moist surfaces meet dry skin, for example the anus. Both the ulcers and the condylomata exude fluid that contains numerous spirochaetes. The infection can be transmitted by contact with these, or with the fluid coming from them.

Following secondary syphilis, the infection usually enters a latent phase. During this stage the infection is entirely silent and the only sign of infection is a positive blood test. Latent syphilis can last for a number of years. Various studies of the natural history of syphilis suggest that between 15 and 40% of people with latent syphilis progress to tertiary syphilis, the rest either spontaneously overcoming the infection or retaining the infection in a dormant form.

Tertiary syphilis usually arises many years after a person becomes infected and it is at this stage that the serious consequences of syphilis can occur. Without treatment, around 20 to 30% of people will die of the complications after being infected for fifteen to twenty years.

The complications of tertiary syphilis can be divided into benign and malignant forms. The main feature of benign tertiary syphilis is known as a gumma. A gumma is an area of inflammatory or allergic response to the presence of the syphilis spirochaetes in the body. The centre of the gumma can become liquified and 'gummy' in texture, hence the name.

The immune response is rarely effective in eradicating the organism or curing the infection and simply causes complications. The inflammatory response of the gumma can gradually expand and can damage those parts of the body that it involves. Gummas can thus affect bone, skin and internal organs and it is the site that becomes involved that determines the symptoms. If bone is affected, fractures may follow relatively minor stresses. If skin is affected, ulcers and sores may develop. If internal organs are involved, there may be no symptoms or there may be serious impairment of organ function and corresponding symptoms. Although gummas are also part of 'benign' tertiary syphilis, depending on what organs they affect, they can behave in a 'malignant' fashion unless treated.

Malignant tertiary syphilis occurs when the infection damages vital organs such as the heart, blood vessels, brain and/or spinal cord. Damage to the brain and spinal cord, is known as neurosyphilis and neurological symptoms result. If the heart and great arteries leading from the heart are damaged, the infection is known as cardiovascular syphilis and cardiac symptoms result.

Neurosyphilis can be further subdivided depending on whether the damage predominantly involves the part of the spinal cord known as the dorsal columns (this complication is called tabes dorsalis) or damage predominantly involves the brain (known as generalised paresis of the insane or GPI). When the damage invoves the spinal cord, the most common symptom is shooting pains and other sensory disturbances particularly in the legs. When the damage predominantly involves the brain, behaviour changes occur. It is not uncommon for these to gradually worsen over a period of many months. Often they are mistaken for psychiatric symptoms and it is only when the psychiatrist tests for syphilis that the diagnosis becomes clear.

Syphilis: Tests and treatment

There are a number of blood tests available for syphilis and, for the inexperienced, they can be a source of confusion. A few simple rules can help to make them more understandable.

There are basically two types of syphilis blood test: non-specific and specific. Both test for antibodies produced by the body in response to the infection.

The antibodies detected by the 'non-specific' test can be produced in response to some other problems too, which partly explains the name. The best known non-specific test is the RPR (Rapid Plasma Reagin) test. The non-specific RPR has two main uses. First, it is a quick, simple screening test. Second, it is a useful indicator of the activity of the infection and can be used to check the response to treatment. A positive RPR needs to be confirmed with a specific test such as the TPHA (Treponaema Pallidum Haem Agglutination test) or the FTA (Fluorescent Treponaema Antibody) test. This is because false positive RPR tests can occur during pregnancy, viral infections, immune diseases and some chronic diseases.

The RPR tends to give high readings when the infection is most active. This characteristic allows it to be used to monitor the success of treatment. Following treatment of syphilis, the RPR should be repeated every three months or so for eighteen months. If the RPR does not drop to a low level over that time or, if it drops but then starts to rise again, the syphilis may not have been cured or reinfection may have occurred. In this case, another course of treatment should be given.

Treatment

The treponaema organism which causes syphilis is always sensitive to penicillin. A prolonged course of penicillin is required which usually involves injections daily for at least ten days.

In people allergic to penicillin, erythromycin or doxycycline can be used.

The RPR reading will decline very gradually if the infection goes untreated for a number of years. A doctor should take this into account when evaluating positive results. It is possible for a person with tertiary syphilis to have a low RPR. In this case further information is needed in order to assess the situation. Details of past treatment and the possibility of reinfection will assist in making the decision about whether the infection is likely to be current and requires re-treatment. Details of the likely duration of infection, neurological symptoms, tests for involvement of the cerebrospinal fluid (CSF) and a chest X-ray will help to evaluate how long treatment should continue. If previous treatment does not seem to have been adequate and tests are consistent with active infection, treatment with penicillin should be given. If the infection has probably been present for more than two years, then a longer course of treatment is indicated. If symptoms suggest tertiary syphilis or if the CSF or chest X-ray findings suggest tertiary syphilis, treatment is probably best given intravenously. This allows larger amounts of penicillin to penetrate the brain and spinal cord. The sudden death of numerous spirochaetes during penicillin treatment can cause a temporary worsening of symptoms. This is known as the 'Herxheimer reaction' and can probably be reduced by giving corticosteroids prior to treatment.

The developing baby is protected from the damaging effects of syphilis infection for about four months after conception. Therefore the diagnosis and treatment of the mother's syphilis in early pregnancy can prevent the devastating effects of inherited syphilis.

AIDS (Aquired Immune Deficiency Syndrome)

AIDS is due to a virus called the *human immunodeficiency virus* (HIV). The virus is so named because it causes immune deficiency by infecting and damaging one of the important cell types responsible for immunity, the body's system of protection from infection. The immune system involves two main types of white blood cell: T cells and B cells. B cells are responsible for producing substances called antibodies that then attack infections. This is known as humoral immunity. T cells are responsible for cells that directly kill infections. This is known as cell-mediated immunity. T cells are

Victor decided to have a checkup at a sexual health clinic because he had not had one for some time, although he had practised safe sex since 1984. After talking to a nurse and a counsellor he decided to have a blood test for HIV, syphilis and hepatitis B.

Two weeks later the test results came back. The HIV test was negative and the hepatitis result was also clear. The nurse suggested a vaccination against hepatitis B, to which Victor agreed.

Victor was shocked to find his last test result, for syphilis, showed a positive RPR test and a positive FTA test. When the nurse asked if he had previously had syphilis, because the RPR result was quite low and was consistent with treated syphilis, Victor said 'No'. The nurse then asked if he could remember ever having had a painless, coin-sized ulcer. After some time, Victor recalled something of the sort in 1982. He had not taken it seriously because it did not seem too nasty.

Based on the test results and Victor's recollections, the nurse concluded that Victor had latent syphilis of some years standing and that he needed treatment to avoid serious complications. Since Victor had a long-standing allergy to penicillin—it made his neck swell and caused breathing difficulties—he was treated for a month with doxycycline and was advised to have blood tests every three to six months for the following two years. The treatment was successful and Victor's syphilis was cured.

divided into helper T cells (T4 or CD4 cells) and suppressor T cells (T8 or CD8 cells). Helper T cells boost the immune response to ensure that an adequate response to infection occurs. Suppressor T cells dampen down the immune response in order to avoid excessive damage. Both of these systems are normally in a very delicate balance which is disrupted by HIV. It can attack the CD4 helper cells, causing a decline in their numbers, and a relative excess of suppressor cells. Immune deficiency then results and the defect in the immune system leaves the infected individual vulnerable to other infections. It is these infections that cause the illness known as AIDS.

AIDS made a dramatic appearance on the world stage during the

1980s but the origin of the virus is unclear and controversial. Some believe it came from Africa, however others have suggested the virus originated in the Americas. However, what really matters is that HIV is now a world-wide problem that we must all face. During the 1980s an enormous amount of research, writing and political debate occurred and several important principles emerged: If the spread of AIDS is to be curbed, steps must be taken to ensure effective prevention, the avoidance of antisocial reactions to people with the infection, and quality care.

HIV can be passed from person to person in three ways. First, through unprotected sexual intercourse where one partner already has the virus. Second, from a mother with HIV to her child during childbirth or during breast feeding. Third, by injecting live virus into the bloodstream. The latter can occur when an individual shares needles and syringes already used by someone with HIV, through needlestick injuries where the needle was recently used for someone

---

Helen and James were involved in a close relationship but before Helen would agree to have sex, she insisted that James be tested for HIV. James felt a little resentful but agreed to have a blood test at the Family Planning Clinic.

Initially, all James wanted to do was to have the blood test and leave. But after talking to the counsellor about the HIV test, other STD tests, and his relationship, James realised there was no point in having a test unless Helen did also, and that they should both take the opportunity to have some other STD tests as well.

After discussions which both felt helped their relationship, they had the recommended tests. Two weeks later, the counsellor saw each of them in turn about their results. They thought it was a little strange that the counsellor wanted to speak to them separately but he explained this was to allow them to speak openly while also protecting their privacy until they were ready to talk together.

The couple had negative HIV test results, but James had a positive chlamydia culture and Helen had some changes in her Pap smear. This was a surprise to both because neither had any symptoms. They agreed to the counsellor making arrangements to have these problems attended to.

with HIV or through blood transfusion using blood from someone with HIV. In Australia, spread through blood transfusions is now very unlikely. Blood donors complete and sign a questionnaire and are asked not to donate blood if there is any suggestion of risk. Furthermore, all blood donations are tested for HIV, hepatitis B, hepatitis C and syphilis before being used. Spread through sexual intercourse and through used needles are the key ways of spreading HIV.

There has been a great deal of debate and misinformation in the media about whether HIV can be spread through heterosexual sex or not. The answer is now known to be emphatically yes. HIV can be spread through any version of sexual intercourse when one partner is infected and the intercourse is unprotected. Indeed, on a world-wide scale, from the earliest days, AIDS was (and still is) predominantly a heterosexual problem. In the worst affected areas of Africa, men and women are known to be infected in equal numbers. This is partly due to a high incidence of other genital infections making people more vulnerable to HIV. These genital infections are not exotic; herpes and chlamydia have been found to play an important role and these are common infections in Western countries too. It seems likely that the key differences between the worst affected areas of the world and some Western countries is that the virus has been present in those areas for longer and has had more time to diffuse widely through the susceptible populations. Also, the virus seems to have been able to spread more widely in areas with high levels of poverty, where prostitution is essential for survival, where treatment of sexually transmitted infections is often unavailable, where condoms are unaffordable and where mass vaccination campaigns depend on reusing needles. In the West, in contrast, sexually transmitted AIDS has been predominantly a problem for gay men, but there seems to be little basis for it staying that way unless prevention is taken seriously by the entire community.

Furthermore, while it is true that HIV can be spread easily through anal intercourse, some people have concluded that vaginal intercourse with someone who may be infected is therefore not a great risk. This is a dangerous example of denial. Similarly, many males seem to need to believe that it is the receptive ('female') partner rather than the insertive ('male') partner who is at risk. In fact, either partner has a significant risk during unprotected anal or vaginal intercourse when the other partner is HIV positive.

It has recently been proposed that the virus can pass from a woman to a man or from a receptive gay man to an insertive gay man by entering the bloodstream through the lining of the urethra via the meatus or eye of the penis. It seems that the cells lining the moist surfaces of the genitals, called dendritic cells, are particularly vulnerable to picking up the virus thus providing a point of entry to the body. It has become clear also that obvious inflammation, abrasions and cuts on the genitals are probably not necessary for the virus to be passed from person to person during intercourse.

Occasionally a few days to weeks after becoming infected with HIV a person will experience an illness similar to the 'flu'. This is known as the seroconversion illness because it typically occurs around the time that the test converts to positive. Usually however, the initial infection with HIV occurs without any symptoms and the infected person can remain well for many years totally unaware that he or she is infected. For reasons that are unclear, after a number of years the virus becomes active and starts to break down the immune system leaving the person vulnerable to particular infections and cancers. These infections are known as opportunistic infections because they take the opportunity to infect people when their defences are low. Likewise, the 'opportunistic' malignancies (cancers) also take the opportunity to develop and spread when the person's defences are weakened. It is these infections and cancers that kill individuals infected with HIV rather than the HIV itself.

It is not until a person's immune system is severely weakened and he or she experiences one of these opportunistic problems that AIDS is said to be occurring. If a person is simply infected with HIV but is not at the stage of having AIDS, then he or she is said to be HIV positive. The average time from infection with HIV to the development of AIDS is around nine years although illness can occur both before or after this period has passed. Around a third to a half of people who have had HIV for nine years will have developed AIDS. The other half to two-thirds will not be so severely affected by this time.

It is not yet certain whether all people who are HIV infected will develop AIDS eventually. During almost all of the nine years after infection except for about the first three months, the HIV test will be positive even if the person is totally symptom free. This is sometimes the source of some confusion: the test usually becomes positive within three months of contracting the virus even though it can take many years to get sick. A positive test indicates that the virus has entered the body and has been intercepted by the body's immune system. The immune system has reacted by producing antibodies and this is what the HIV antibody test or 'AIDS test' detects. This is why a person who has a positive test is said to be 'HIV positive' or 'antibody positive'. All positive tests are checked with a supplementary test called a 'western blot'. A western blot test allows the antibodies to be examined more precisely in order to differentiate false positive tests from true positive HIV tests. Only tests that are confirmed with western blotting are reported by the lab as positive. It is wise for doctors to test another blood sample if a test is found to be positive, just to ensure that there was not a mixup or mistake.

Although the immune system produces antibodies in response to the virus entering the bloodstream, HIV has special properties that allow it to avoid being destroyed by the immune system. Unlike many other infections, the presence of antibodies indicates ongoing infection with HIV rather than past resolved infection. Because the virus has an unusual ability to avoid destruction by the immune system, the infection lasts for life. Hence, the virus can be passed to others during unsafe sex or via needles virtually from the time that infection occurs. If the virus is passed on, the person who picks it up and becomes HIV positive has a chance of developing AIDS even before the person who was first infected with HIV. For most of the nine or so years of the infection most people show little or no sign of ill-health and are usually unrecognisable from uninfected people. Precautions should therefore apply to everyone regardless of whether they have been tested and regardless of the result.

Elisa AIDS test detects HIV-1 only, not HIV-2 (African)

Preventing the spread of HIV

Avoiding HIV can be complex and precautions need to be tailor-made to each individual although some general rules apply. The main ways of preventing HIV infection are to prevent the virus from being passed on during sex and by needles containing blood. There are numerous preventive strategies all of which will protect against infection. It is important to understand them and use whichever precaution(s) is best suited to an individual situation. Avoiding intercourse is one way of being safe. Remember that it is a person's right to say no. Saying no to intercourse does not necessarily mean saying no to any form of sexual pleasure. Prevention is much more likely to be successful if some sort of sexual 'outlet' is permitted. Be creative, sex can sometimes lose its value if intercourse is all there is to it. Mutual masturbation is a common way of giving pleasure while still being safe. Kissing, caressing and massage are all safe.

On the other hand, if intercourse is an essential part of a person's sex life, there is no choice but to make sure that a condom is used. Condoms used properly are an effective way of stopping HIV. Many people make a lot of fuss about the fact that condoms can fail. In fact condoms do have a failure rate but this depends almost entirely on the person using the condom. In the hands of people who have a clear understanding of how condoms work and how to use them, their failure rate is extremely low. It is probably best for a person to tell his or her partner that condoms are always going to be used at the beginning of the relationship, and to make sure they are always handy. It is also important to practise condom use on one's own before using them for sex.

Most studies showing condoms to be an imperfect method for preventing pregnancy are open to criticism because the people taking part probably were not too worried about avoiding becoming pregnant. There have also been many studies that show that condoms used properly do stop HIV. The bottom line is that the failure rate of condoms is probably not as high as the failure rate of monogamy (that is, having one sexual partner). Furthermore, if people use condoms consistently and, as a result, the virus remains at a low level in a population, then occasional failures of condom usage will not expose the person to a substantial risk (if any) of contracting HIV. Monogamy is often more complex than appears on the surface. An individual seeking assurances that he or she is not infected with HIV must first be certain that his/her partner is not HIV positive and is not likely to become positive. In short he or she must be sure that the partner has not or will not share needles and also has only ever had one partner. Similarly sexual abstinence also has a significant failure rate: abstinence would seem to be the domain of a few special religious people and is therefore not generally useful for stopping STD spread.

Preventing sexual spread of HIV is only half the story. A major means of HIV spread, particularly in Western countries, is through shared needles and syringes. Again, precautions should be tailor-made to the individual case. Some people will be able to give up drugs. Others will be able to change to non-injectable drugs. Others will not yet be able to give drugs up or may continue to use them on an occasional or 'recreational' basis. In this case, the buzz word is 'harm minimisation'. Harm minimisation means teaching people

---

Mos had a difficult adolescence full of questions about where he was heading and what he was worth. As he got older he discovered he could get more attention if he was considered an extrovert and it wasn't long before he had a reputation as a real 'rager'.

Occasionally at parties he would shoot up with speed (injectable amphetamines) and once he even had a taste of smac or hammer (injectable heroin). The first time he 'used' he didn't have a needle, so he took a chance and shared someone else's 'fit' (needle and syringe). As he became more used to using, he always made sure he had a small sachet of bleach in his car to clean syringes.

One day a friend talked him into getting a HIV test and the clinic advisor also suggested that consistent use of clean needles and syringes was safer than bleach. He thought about this and agreed to take a supply. The advisor said that the police did not hassle people just because they had syringes.

A fortnight later, Mos was told his HIV test was positive. This triggered a 'big drift'. Why make plans? What about his family? Would he tell his favourite sister? He really needed to but if he did, would her husband ever let him near his niece and nephew who meant so much to him?

After holding everything in for a while, it finally got too much and he decided to call the AIDS Help Line. He even thought about saying he was going to suicide. Once he was talking and before he knew what had happened, he was engulfed by a flood of tears. After a long talk, he decided to see his advisor who helped him gradually pull his life together.

He decided to tell all the members of his family and found they were marvellous. Everyone was upset, but they all much preferred to know and help. Mos also joined a support group where he could talk to others similarly affected. He couldn't believe how good he started to feel about such a difficult situation .

who continue to use drugs to do so as safely as possible. Providing sterile needles and syringes (through needle exchange programs, for example) and a safe method for their disposal has been shown to be effective. Alternatively, needles and syringes should be cleaned between use, when sterile ones are not available. The 2×2×2 method is the most popular way of doing this. In this method the fit (needle and syringe) is rinsed twice in water to rinse out any blood. It is then rinsed twice in bleach to disinfect the interior. Finally the syringe is rinsed twice in fresh water to rinse out residual bleach.

A four-pronged approach to dealing with HIV

The first approach to dealing with HIV is prevention, all too often overlooked in modern medicine. Prevention is paramount if AIDS is to be controlled.

The second approach is relevant when a person is HIV positive but has no symptoms or signs of the infection. In this case the main priority is to keep that person in good health and where possible to improve it. Nutrition, social supports, treating other infections, vaccinating against hepatitis and flu, counselling and monitoring the immune system are all important. At this stage, the immune system may or may not be severely damaged. The most useful way of checking immune function is to take a sample of blood and CD4 cell count (also known as the T cell count). This test provides a guide to the total number of CD4 cells per millilitre of blood. If the immune system is normal, then prevention of HIV spread to others, maintaining health and treating symptoms are key objectives. If the immune system is mildly affected (CD4 cells less than 500/cubic mm) the infected person should consider antiviral treatment such as azidothymidine (AZT), dideoxyinosine (DDI) or dideoxycytidine (DDC) in order to reduce any further damage. If the immune system is severely damaged (CD4 cells less than 200/cubic mm) medications (such as cotrimoxazole) to prevent opportunistic complications are appropriate.

The third approach applies when the person develops symptoms even though he or she may not be unwell enough to be regarded as having AIDS. Here too prevention of further spread and maintenance of good health are very important. But controlling symptoms is also a priority. Even the development of minor symptoms can be frightening and care should involve careful explanation and checking for serious causes. Reassurance may be all that is needed, but sometimes medications to relieve annoying but non-serious symptoms are also required. Again, if the immune system is mildly depressed, antiviral medications may be indicated. If the immunity is seriously depressed, medications to prevent opportunistic infections should be taken. Do not fall into the trap of attributing all symptoms of ill-health to HIV/AIDS. Some individuals who are not even HIV positive become obsessed with symptoms that they are convinced are due to HIV infection. Often general public information on AIDS contains a comprehensive list of symptoms that may be associated with AIDS and often these are unclear and sound similar to those that everybody experiences from time to time.

The fourth approach to dealing with HIV occurs when severely depressed immune function occurs and an opportunistic infection or opportunistic malignancy develops. At this point, when the infected person is said to have AIDS, it is unlikely that the damage to the immune system can be reversed. Over the next couple of years, periods of stable health are typically punctuated by episodes of opportunistic illness every few months. Each of these episodes makes in-roads on health and the risk to life itself becomes evident. Appropriate strategies at this point include measures to improve general health, treatment of symptoms, administration of medications that will prevent opportunistic infections, use of antiviral drugs to reduce the activity of HIV, and diagnosis and treatment of opportunistic conditions. At this point too, support from friends, family, lovers and health carers becomes critically important. Often quality of life can be greatly improved by explanation and steps which enable the person to make his or her own decisions about what tests and treatments are necessary. Helping the person to understand what is happening and giving him or her as much control as possible are important components of care. Prevention of the spread of HIV through sex, drugs or hospital accidents remains vital.

Strategies to improve general health include good, balanced, calorie-rich nutrition, treatment of treatable infections, and counselling and support aimed at coming to terms with AIDS and developing a positive outlook. Drugs can be administered to prevent the pneumonia commonly associated with AIDS, known as pneumocystis pneumonia. This previously common complication of AIDS often caused death, but treatment is improving. Prevention can be

Claire is an active member of the AIDS Council. She often visits schools and teaches about AIDS—particularly how to prevent its spread. She is driven by the hope that others won't end up in her sitaution.

Sometimes she feels angry about the widespread lack of consideration for women with AIDS including herself. She also finds that many people cannot separate their anti-gay mentality from a more just approach that emphasises unconditional care and effective, genuine prevention.

Claire knows a lot about AIDS and keeps a close eye on her immune status and her nutritional needs. She also realises the importance of getting sound psychological support. She is happy in the knowledge that she is doing as much as she can to maintain her health and that everything seems to be in control.

achieved by a variety of medications including dapsone or cotri-moxazole tablets (Septrin or Bactrim).

Antiviral drugs such as AZT, DDI and DDC are also increasingly useful. Previously AZT was used in high dose to treat illness and, used this way, it often caused side-effects. Now AZT is used in low dosage at an earlier stage to prevent damage to the immune system. Using this approach, side-effects are much less common. The main problem with AZT is that over a couple of years, HIV tends to develop resistance to it and its effect wears off. New strategies are now being developed to overcome this problem. The key strategy is to develop a combination of drugs used in low doses to suppress the virus. It is hoped that this will reduce side-effects and that drugs given in combination will prevent resistance. The outlook for success using these strategies is promising and it is hoped that over the next few years a combination of medications will be developed that will suppress the virus indefinitely. The current task is to keep people well enough to benefit from these developments. Nevertheless, a cure is still not in sight and prevention of infection is far preferable.

Opportunistic complications of AIDS

Opportunitic illnesses in AIDS are complex but are included here because people often want to know about AIDS in great detail.

Opportunistic infections only occur when the immune system is impaired. Most infections do not pose a threat to people with normal immunity and rather than being caught from others are usually the result of the reactivation of past infections due to poor immunity. Because of immune system deficiency, treatment with antibiotics often only suppresses the opportunistic infection rather than cures it. As a result, life-long treatment may be necessary. Common opportunistic infections include pneumocystis pneumonia, cerebral toxoplasmosis, atypical mycobacteria, cryptococcal meningitis, CMV retinitis and cryptosporidium diarrhoea.

Pneumocystis pneumonia is caused by a parasitic infection that infects the lungs of most people early in life. It lies dormant for as long as the immune system operates normally. When CD4 cells are severely depressed, pneumocystis can reactivate and cause a pneumonia. If the CD4 cells decline in number, medications such as dapsone, cotrimoxazole or pentamidine can be given to prevent pneumonia. If pneumonia occurs, it causes the development of fever and shortness of breath. Diagnosis is based on a chest X-ray and an examination of sputum from deep in the lungs (induced sputum). It is necessary to examine induced sputum because the cough is usually dry. Induced sputum is obtained by inhaling a mist of saline and then coughing it up for testing. Treatment with an oxygen mask if necessary, antibiotics and corticosteroids has been found to be effective.

Cerebral toxoplasmosis is due to a parasitic infection called *Toxoplasma gondii*. This is often aquired during childhood and lies dormant for as long as the immune system functions properly. If CD4 cell numbers drop well below 200 per cubic mm, the toxoplasma can reactivate. If it reactivates in the brain, then a brain abscess can develop resulting in a progressive worsening of brain symptoms. The diagnosis is made with a CT brain scan and by confirming past infection by testing for toxoplasma antibodies in blood. Treatment with antibiotics—for example: sulphonamides and pyrimethamine—can prove life-saving. Life-long antibiotics are usually necessary to prevent recurrences.

Atypical mycobacteria (MAI) are related to the bacteria that cause tuberculosis (TB). These bacteria cause a widespread infection of the blood. Typical symptoms include unrelenting, progressive weight loss, fevers and drenching night sweats. Diagnosis involves a culture of blood for these bacteria in a special tube. Treatment with a combination of drugs usually reserved for TB has been effective.

Cytomegalovirus (CMV) is a common type of viral infection that affects up to 60% of the general population. In most people it causes a mild or symptom-free infection. This typically lies dormant but, again, if immune function declines the infection can reactivate and cause problems such as damage to the back of the eye (retina) with progressive loss of vision. Diagnosis involves examination of the retina through an ophthalmoscope for typical CMV damage. A blood test for antibodies can confirm past infection and identify CMV as a possible cause of eye problems.

Cryptococcus is a fungus that can cause infection in the layers around the brain (meningitis). Progressively worsening headache over a week or more is the main feature. Diagnosis can be made by testing blood for cryptococcal antigen and by performing a spinal tap. A spinal tap or lumbar puncture involves inserting a needle into the fluid surrounding the spinal cord and taking a sample of the fluid. The fluid is called cerebrospinal fluid or CSF. The CSF is examined under the microscope and cultured for infections. Treatment of cryptococcal meningitis involves antibiotics such as amphotericin or fluconazole. In people with AIDS, this treatment is usually life-long.

Cryptosporidium is a parasite that can cause severe, relentless watery diarrhoea (cryptosporidium is completely different from cryptococcus). The diagnosis is made by examining a specimen of the diarrhoea for the organism with a microscope and using special staining techniques. Effective treatment is not yet known although new drugs are currently being developed.

Apart from the opportunitic infections, the other problem that affects people with AIDS is the opportunistic malignancies or cancers. These include a previously unusual cancer of the small blood channels called **Kaposi's sarcoma** (KS) and a cancer of the white blood cells called **B cell lymphoma**. Normally the immune system patrols the body and detects cancers early and eliminates them. When the immune system is depressed these cancers can develop more easily. KS causes red-purple raised firm nodules on the skin and internal organs. Ensuring good nutrition and improving general health is usually helpful. Radiotherapy can help to shrink troublesome areas and a drug called interferon alpha can improve skin KS. Both lymphoma and KS can be confirmed by biopsy. This involves taking a tiny sample of the discoloured area for examination under the microscope. Sometimes chemotherapy also becomes necessary although this approach has had mixed success.

Another blood borne infection deserves mention in this chapter— **Epstein-Barr virus** (EBV). It belongs to the herpes family of viruses but has a very different pattern of infection from the herpes simplex virus.

EBV can be spread in saliva, is often symptom-free and remains in the body for life. It infects the throat and a type of white blood cell called a B cell causing a sore throat, swollen glands and fever— thus the name 'glandular fever'. Once infected, an individual carries EBV for life but it is unclear whether the virus can cause further symptoms after the initial infection has settled. About a third of the population carries EBV.

Exposure to EBV can be confirmed by antibody tests. A positive total antibody test indicates contact and subsequent carriage but gives no indication as to when the contact occurred. A positive IgM test indicates recent infection. The test for EBV is known as a monospot test or a Paul-Bunnell test. Positive tests do not necessarily imply that the infection is causing any symptoms or disease. That is a clinical diagnosis.

EBV is occasionally associated with serious complications including cancer of the pharynx (throat) and lymphoma (cancer of white blood cells). These complications are rare and seem to occur in particular populations. Cancer of the throat is restricted to some South-East Asian people while lymphoma occasionally occurs in people with very poor immunity such as people with AIDS.

Conclusion

A number of infections can be transmitted by intimate sexual contact and yet cause little or no disease of the genitals. The most important of these are HIV, hepatitis and syphilis. All can be silent for prolonged periods and all can cause serious long term consequences. Diagnosis is almost always confirmed by blood tests although the question as to which test to use and how to interpret the tests is often a source of confusion. Syphilis has become uncommon in the West, however, it has not disappeared. Treatment is very easy, with penicillin the most effective treatment. Hepatitis B is preventable and people who are likely to be at risk should be vaccinated. Nowadays, the prevention of HIV is also paramount and a sophisticated approach to teaching safe sexual practices is essential. Safety needs to be tailor-made to the individual but a few key rules apply. The age old approach of ignorance, denial and folk-lore are no longer acceptable. Effective prevention rather than its token acknowledgement is vital. Western medicine has been weak in the areas of education and prevention in the past but this must change. High quality care for individuals with HIV/AIDS is crucial. Discrimination and prejudice are not civilised nor acceptable. Compassion, support and care are bare basics and should not be seen as a luxury. Safe sex, safe drug use and universal precautions in health-care settings are the inescapable 'new facts of life'. The greatest caring act is to help to prevent infection in the first place.

Chapter Nine

STDs AND SEXUAL HEALTH

The full orchestra of male and female reproductive parts and processes need to be working for maintenance of fertility.

On the male side, the testicles must be making adequate numbers of healthy sperm, the system of tubes and tubules intact, and the penis capable of erection, vaginal penetration and ejaculation. The sperm must then negotiate the vagina, cervix and uterine cavity and pass into a Fallopian tube.

On the female side, at least one of the Fallopian tubes must be free from blockage or malfunction and must have capably performed the job of capturing an egg released from an ovary. This in turn relies on a well-functioning menstrual cycle that has ensured the production of a mature egg with appropriate hormone support.

Fertilisation, the fusing of sperm and egg to create the beginnings of a new human life, must also go to plan.

Scientists examining the earliest stages of human life have established that the first contact between egg and sperm usually occurs in the section of Fallopian tube nearest the ovary. Although several hundred sperm may surround the egg at this stage, usually just one enters it. As soon as this happens, a chemical signal passes from the egg to its tough elastic outer membrane, ensuring no further sperm penetrate. Occasionally, more than one sperm gets in, resulting in an abnormal embryo that will not survive.

The fertilised egg remains in the Fallopian tube for two or three days, dividing repeatedly as it slowly journeys towards the uterus. It is important to realise that the Fallopian tube is not merely a neutral channel for this important journey. It provides essential assistance.

First, the Fallopian tube releases substances that create a favourable environment for continued survival of the fertilised egg. Second, the millions of tiny hairs called cilia that line its inner surface, like

104

the pile of a shag rug, beat constantly towards the uterus. As well, the muscles of the Fallopian tube contract periodically, giving the fertilised egg a gentle push in the right direction.

What causes ectopic pregnancies?

If the Fallopian tube is blocked or otherwise damaged, or the cilia are not working properly, the fertilised egg may never reach the uterus and may start to grow within the tube.

The result is a tubal or ectopic pregnancy ('ectopic' meaning not in the right place). If this occurs, the embryo eventually has no room to grow and this can cause bleeding and/or pain. If a large volume of blood is lost, rarely, death of the woman and the embryo may result.

Fortunately, the problem is usually diagnosed and treated before any irreparable damage is done. A doctor may suspect an ectopic pregnancy when an ultrasound scan fails to show any evidence of a pregnancy in the uterus, yet a woman has a positive pregnancy test. Surgery is still the usual procedure for removing an ectopic pregnancy, but this can now frequently be done down an endoscope (laparoscopy—see below) thus avoiding major surgery. Recent studies suggest that the same result may be achieved faster, more easily and more economically in the future with an injectable treatment.

Pelvic inflammatory disease (PID)

Some STDs have the potential to damage the Fallopian tubes, thereby reducing the likelihood of an egg entering them, or sperm ever meeting the egg or, if fertilisation does occur, of the embryo ever reaching the receptive environment of the uterus.

The umbrella term for infection of the internal sex organs, as noted previously, is **'pelvic inflammatory disease' (PID)**. STDs are not the only cause, but they are the major factor in a significant number of cases.

Swedish research indicates that STDs pose a powerful threat to female fertility. If 100 women have a single attack of PID, 11 are likely to become infertile. Of 100 women who have two attacks, 23 will be rendered infertile. And after three attacks among 100 women, an alarming 54 will be infertile.

In a similar way, a man's fertility can be affected by STD-induced damage to the organs in which sperm are produced, transported or stored. For example, untreated **gonorrhoea** can result in obstruction of the vas deferens, thereby preventing the outflow of sperm from the testicles.

Just as PID is a significant cause of fertility problems in women, it is also a major cause of fertility impairment in men. The damaging effects of infection may take longer to become obvious in men than women because men produce millions of sperm in a single ejaculate whereas women typically produce a single mature egg each month.

Causes and treatments of PID in women

PID incorporates inflammation of the uterus (**endometritis**), the Fallopian tubes (**salpingitis**) and the lining of the pelvic organs (**pelvic peritonitis**). Once an infection is established in the Fallopian tubes, the infective material (pus) can leak into the abdomen causing peritonitis.

Although PID is usually caused by organisms such as *Neisseria gonorrhoeae* or *Chlamydia trachomatis* which pass into the vagina during intercourse, pelvic infection can sometimes follow appendicitis, pelvic surgery or miscarriage.

The infection usually starts in the cervix and then spreads to the endometrium and Fallopian tubes. Once inflammation develops, other organisms which usually live harmlessly in the vagina may take advantage of the new situation, becoming secondary invaders and adding to the damage caused by the initial problem organism.

The uterus and Fallopian tubes are moderately well protected from infectious organisms by a plug of thick mucus in the cervix that acts like a door impairing their passage for most of the menstrual cycle. Taking the Pill thickens this mucus and makes the barrier better. However this protection is far from perfect and during menstruation and early in the menstrual cycle, the mucus is relatively sparse, making the uterus and Fallopian tubes more accessible to bacteria.

PID often has no symptoms, yet major damage to fertility may silently occur. If you have had sex with several partners and you are unsure about whether you may have contracted an infection, it is important to ask your doctor to check for gonorrhoea and chlamydia. And if your partner develops any infections, make sure you are checked and treated too.

Some women develop symptoms such as a tingling or burning sensation when passing urine or an unusual vaginal discharge. If any such symptoms occur, it is important to see a doctor immediately and have them checked out.

If an infection progresses to PID, symptoms may include lower abdominal pain and tenderness, deep pain when having sex, menstrual disturbances and/or fever. Sometimes PID also occurs without any symptoms at all.

Both chlamydia and gonococcus organisms can also cause infection of the urethra (the tube from the bladder through which urine passes to the outside) in men and women, causing pain on passing urine.

Although pain in the pelvis may have other causes, it is important to check for PID promptly to minimise the chance of permanent fertility impairment.

Treatment is usually simple and effective—a course of antibiotics in the form of tablets or capsules or sometimes injections. It is very important to take the full course of treatment prescribed and not to have unprotected sex until you have finished. It is also important to contact any partner who may also have been infected so that he or she can be checked and treated too—otherwise you may be reinfected or someone else may become infected.

A barrier to early treatment is the lack of a simple method for diagnosing female PID conclusively. A doctor cannot easily examine the organs involved as they lie deep in the pelvis.

A procedure called laparoscopy can do the job, but it requires a general anaesthetic and a small incision below the belly button. Gynaecologists use the laparoscope, a magnifying instrument with its own light, to inspect the abdominal cavity, the uterus, Fallopian tubes and ovaries. A special probe is usually inserted through an incision in the abdomen to allow the doctor to grasp or move the pelvic organs, thus enabling a more complete inspection.

If PID is present, its severity is quickly evident. In mild cases, the laparoscope reveals a reddening of the tubes. In more severe cases, the tubes may appear swollen and puffy due to a build-up of fluid related to the inflammation. In severe instances of PID, the tubes are blocked and are full of pus (**pyosalpinx**).

Laparoscopy enables inspection of the outside of the tubes and allows major degrees of damage to be detected but it cannot accurately assess the changes of the inner lining. A new technique called falloposcopy has recently been developed which enables the inside of the tubes to be checked using an 0.4mm diameter flexible telescope. The use of this technique will help assess the condition of the tubes after an episode of STD.

Risk factors for PID

Women are most at risk after childbirth, miscarriage, surgery to the reproductive organs and abortion. In such situations, organisms that normally inhabit the vagina without causing any problem may multiply and cause harm.

The type of contraception a woman uses may also alter her risk of PID. Inflammation of the Fallopian tubes and uterus may be aggravated by an IUD (intra uterine contraceptive device) which acts as a foreign body and may make it easier for invasion by bacteria. Women with other risk factors for PID should not use this method of contraception.

On the other hand, both the combined Pill (that is, standard oral contraception) and the progestogen-only Pill (the Mini-Pill) decrease the risk of PID. This occurs because they make it more difficult for bacteria as well as sperm to penetrate the cervical mucus. They are not adequate protection against STDs on their own, however.

Diaphragms restrict the passage of bacteria and perhaps some viruses also, and spermicides are toxic to many micro-organisms. Once again, they are not adequate as the sole protection against STDs.

The condom is considered the best barrier against bacterial and viral STDs as well as being a reliable contraceptive when used consistently and correctly.

It is rare for women or men to get PID unless they are sexually active. Having sex with different partners or having a regular partner who has sex with a number of other partners greatly increases the risk of a chlamydial or gonococcal infection which can cause PID.

Even taking into account factors such as these, younger women appear to be more at risk of PID than comparable older women. The reasons for this are not yet clear.

Once a woman has had one episode of PID, the chances of a later episode are considerably greater. This is probably due both to the persistence of a small number of harmful organisms despite treatment and to the vulnerability of damaged tissues to later bacterial invasion.

PID prevention

Prevention of PID is something every woman and man should know about.

As noted previously, condoms are the most effective protection against genital infections. If used properly, there is very little risk of infections being transmitted.

A diaphragm may also decrease the chances of sexually transmitted infections spreading to the cervix, but it is nowhere near as effective as a condom.

Both condoms and diaphragms used with spermicides, available from local pharmacies, are more effective against STDs as the chemicals they contain can inactivate some of the harmful organisms.

Finally, while limiting your number of partners reduces your risk of coming into contact with infection, remember that intercourse even once without protection is enough for transmission. The healthy good looks of a partner and all the assurances of being safe in the past offer no reliable guarantee.

Causes and treatment of PID in men

The most common symptom of **PID in men** is the symptom of passing pins and needles when urinating. STDs which cause **urethritis**, inflammation of the urethra, often cause this unpleasant sensation. Inflammation of the testicles (**orchitis**) causing pain, or inflammation of the prostate (**prostatitis**) can result from some infections. Other symptoms remote from the site of infection, eg. conjunctivitis, or arthritis may be caused by some infections, and the occurrence of rashes has previously been described.

Finally, it has to be remembered that some STDs cause no symptoms at all. These can silently cause damage and can be inadvertently passed on to others.

The treatment of PID consists of eradicating the infective organism after its identification in appropriate cultures.

The impact of STDs on pregnancy and newborn

During pregnancy, the blood of the fetus passes through the placenta (afterbirth) which is separated from the mother's blood by a thin layer of cells.

Many substances and some organisms such as viruses and bacteria can move across this thin barrier during the course of the pregnancy, and thus circulate through the fetus, sometimes causing infection leading to possible damage. The result may be an abnormality in fetal development, miscarriage, premature labour or even death of the fetus with subsequent stillbirth.

Syphilis was the first organism recognised to be transmissible during pregnancy from maternal to fetal blood. Infection of the fetus by the spirochaetes of syphilis can cause miscarriage during the middle three months of pregnancy. It can also result in the birth of a child with serious developmental abnormalities of the face, teeth, joints, hearing and vision.

When it was recognised that these abnormalities did not develop until about sixteen weeks of pregnancy, the importance of early intervention to treat the infection in pregnant women became obvious.

Every pregnant woman should ideally be tested for syphilis during her first antenatal medical check. This practice can virtually eliminate the birth defects associated with syphilis.

Among the most recently discovered and most sinister STDs which can be transmitted via maternal blood during pregnancy is the AIDS virus, HIV. About one in every three babies born to women who are HIV positive are found to be infected with HIV after birth. Unfortunately, unlike syphilis, there is no known treatment to prevent infection of the baby during pregnancy, nor is it clear why some babies and not others become infected.

The same can be said about hepatitis B, another blood-borne infection that can be transmitted during pregnancy.

A further opportunity for infection by STD organisms inhabiting the vagina or cervix occurs when the fetus passes through the birth canal during a vaginal delivery.

The transmission of infections in this way has been recognised for many years and is the reason for wiping the eyes of every newborn baby with silver nitrate immediately after delivery. The target in this case is gonorrhoea which can cause a severe inflammation of eye tissue and subsequent blindness. Chlamydia can also be transmitted during birth. To prevent chlamydia-induced eye damage or pneumonia in newborn babies, appropriate antibiotics are prescribed. Mothers may receive them to treat the genital infection before delivery if the infection is diagnosed in time, and babies may receive them after birth to prevent or treat the eye infection and pneumonia.

Herpes is another infection that can be transmitted during childbirth and that can result in widespread infection and subsequent death. Babies who become infected in this way can develop symptoms of severe brain damage during their second week of life and they run a 50:50 chance of dying as a result. Recent advances in early detection and treatment of herpes in pregnant women has improved the situation markedly.

Treating mothers with STDs during pregnancy must be undertaken with great care as some of the usual antibiotic therapies are harmful to the developing baby. For example, tetracyclines which are used to treat chlamydia can cause maldevelopment of the bones and teeth and therefore should be avoided. Penicillin and erythromycin are considered to be among the safest of the antibiotics and hence are often used to treat gonorrhoea, syphilis and chlamydia during pregnancy. The correct choice of antibiotic is of critical importance and input from an experienced medical practitioner is essential.

Unfortunately, antibiotics do not kill viruses such as herpes, hepatitis and HIV.

Cancer of the cervix and its early forms; the importance of the Pap smear

In the past, abnormalities of the cells of the cervix were called dysplasia. Today, they are referred to as **Cervical Intraepithelial Neoplasia (CIN)** which reflects current thinking that they may be early forms (precursors) of cervix cancer.

Screening for cell abnormalities using Pap smears has been available for several decades and has proved effective in suggesting possible irregularities at an early stage when treatment is likely to be successful.

By encouraging women to have Pap smears every second year from the time sexual activity starts, it is possible to identify early stage abnormalities effectively and economically and then to offer curative treatment. Pap smears every two years are an important way that women can protect themselves from cancer of the cervix which, if left untreated, can invade other tissues and may eventually cause death.

There is good evidence that pre-cancerous abnormalities of the cervix are associated with sexual activity, possibly via infectious organisms transferred during sexual contact. Research suggests that certain strains of the wart virus, also known as *Human Papilloma Virus (HPV)*, are involved, specifically HPV types 16, 18, 31 and perhaps 33. The majority of HPV changes to cells are of no significance and spontaneously regress. However, under the right conditions, types 16, 18, 31 and possibly 33 may result in CIN, which may in turn progress to cancer of the cervix.

HPV infections have long been recognised as the cause of genital warts. About two out of three people who have sexual contact with a person infected with the wart virus will themselves show signs of infection within a few months or years. Although external genital warts are clearly visible on the penis or vulva, HPV infection of the cervix is not always visible to the naked eye. Invisible or subclinical HPV infection is diagnosed by the characteristic appearance of cells obtained from the cervix during a Pap smear, or a colposcopy (see below).

The cells which show abnormal changes occur first at the junction between the glandular and skin-type lining of the cervix. This area is known as the transformation zone because of the characteristic cell type found there.

Before taking a Pap smear, the cervix is examined. This is achieved with the help of an instrument called a vaginal speculum which allows inspection of the cervix by separating the front and back walls of the vagina.

A special brush and a fine wooden spatula are then used to take a sample of cells painlessly from the transformation zone. These cells are smeared on to a glass slide and examined under a microscope after appropriate treatment with a chemical fixative and the application of a stain.

Wart-like change, CIN, or fully-developed cancer can then be detected. If a Pap smear suggests any of these abnormalities, further examination is necessary.

The next step is usually colposcopy which enables assessment of the site from which the abnormal cells came, the nature and severity of the abnormality and the extent of the problem. Colposcopy is an examination with a special magnifying microscope (a colposcope) that resembles a pair of binoculars on a stand. Prior to the examination, the cervix is cleansed with acetic acid and stained with iodine to highlight any abnormal areas. It is a painless procedure, the only discomfort arising from the use of the vaginal speculum.

It is also possible to take a sample of a small area of the cervix (a biopsy) so that the abnormality can be examined in detail under the microscope. This allows more accurate assessment of any suspicious areas found on the Pap smear and/or on colposcopy.

Treatment to destroy any abnormal cells can begin once the nature of the abnormality, its site and extent, have been determined.

Several approaches are used, depending on the type of problem detected. Sometimes it is possible to remove the offending tissue using an electric current (diathermy) or a laser. All have high cure rates. It is very rare for more major surgery to be required.

Occasionally, if the whole of the abnormal area is not clearly visible on colposcopic examination, a small area of tissue (called a cone biopsy) is taken. This can be done using a scalpel, diathermy or laser.

Hysterectomy is rarely necessary but may be called for if the CIN has progressed to invasive cancer.

Ongoing surveillance with regular Pap smears is essential to ensure the problem does not recur. Initially, smears may be carried out every three to six months, and then at yearly intervals.

In the state of Victoria during 1990, over 400,000 women had a Pap smear, but seven out of ten women most at risk of cervix cancer did not come forward to be tested. Reassuringly, eight out of every ten smears done were completely normal or showed changes considered to be insignificant. Less than four in every 100 smears showed CIN changes and only one in every 2000 smears suggested a possible cancer of the cervix.

Sexual dysfunction following STD diagnosis

Most people are distressed to find they have an STD.

However, most cope with the diagnosis and, after appropriate treatment, resume a normal life including an active sex life.

A minority of people experience on-going psychological problems and may complain of a loss of interest in sex, impotence (the inability to have an erection in men), or an inability to enjoy sex or to reach a climax (anorgasmia). In such situations, input from a sexual health counsellor may prove helpful.

The STD checkup

It is natural to feel somewhat nervous and hesitant about having a medical checkup for a possible STD.

This section aims to make things a little easier for you by outlining what you can expect to happen.

You may choose to have the examination at your local medical clinic, a student health centre, a Family Planning Clinic or a specialised sexual health/STD service.

What happens first in an STD checkup?

When you arrive for your appointment, you will probably be asked to fill out a short questionnaire which will include details of your name, address, date of birth and occupation. While these details (and all later findings) are confidential, most STD clinics are happy for you to withhold details if you desire.

Some clinics will ask you to complete a further questionnaire about your medical history. Otherwise a doctor or nurse will discuss with you any current or previous medical problems or symptoms such as an unusual discharge, rash, lump or bump. You will also be asked for details of any medications you are taking and the nature of any surgical procedures you have had. You will probably also be asked some questions about your sexual partner(s) and sexual practices in order to obtain a clear idea about your STD risk.

In addition, a woman having an STD-related examination is likely to be asked for details of her menstrual pattern, at what age she started having periods, whether her periods are painful, how regularly they occur, what sort of contraception she is using, if any, and previous pregnancies and/or abortions.

Questions to men will cover any unusual symptoms they have noticed, especially a penile discharge, discomfort on passing urine, or the presence of any rash, ulcer, lump or sore. Any generalised symptoms such as lethargy, tiredness, hot sweats, lack of appetite, weight loss, or change of bowel habits will be noted, as will details of sexual history.

Doctors working in this area are usually sensitive to the anxiety-provoking nature of the visit and will do their best to make you feel at ease. Remember that *you* have a say in who will treat you. It is very important to choose a doctor who you feel you can trust and who gives honest and complete answers.

What happens during the physical examination (women)?

The physical examination typically starts with a blood pressure check and the doctor may examine your breasts for lumps. The doctor will then look at your abdomen before proceeding to an examination of the genital organs, starting with an inspection of the vulva and then the vagina and cervix. To enable a view of the internal organs, an instrument called a speculum will be used to separate the labia majora and minora. The doctor will usually warm and moisten it and, if you can relax when it is inserted, the examination will be easier. By pushing your bottom down into the couch, the muscles of the vagina will relax more. It may also help to make two fists with your hands and place them under your bottom to tilt your pelvis. Some women are keen to observe the examination and, if this applies to you, ask the doctor to provide a mirror.

If the doctor wants to check what organisms are present in the vagina and cervix, he or she will take swabs as described in previous chapters.

Some of the vaginal secretions may also be removed by a small suction device. This is necessary for certain types of test which require samples in droplet form, for example for trichomonas.

When examining the cervix, the doctor checks specifically for any discharge or inflammation (redness). If a Pap smear is in order, the doctor will take a sample of cells from the cervix for examination by a specialist cytologist.

Computer systems for recording the results of all Pap smears have recently been established in some Australian states, some operated by government agencies and others by private pathology enterprises. This ensures that new tests can be interpreted in the light of previous results, women can be reminded by letter if they are overdue for a smear and the memories of doctors jogged if they have not followed up on an abnormal finding. As with all systems, results may be overlooked occasionally, so take it upon yourself to ring the clinic where the test was taken to find out your results.

The doctor may also take swabs from blisters on the vulva and collect scrapings from any rash that is evident. An anal examination may also be indicated.

All samples collected will be examined by the doctor or by a pathology laboratory.

In most cases, the doctor will also perform a bimanual examination. This involves the placement of two fingers inside the vagina while the fingers of the other hand are placed on the lower abdomen. The procedure may feel uncomfortable but not painful. It allows the doctor to gain a good idea of the size and shape of the uterus, any evidence of tenderness or thickening of the Fallopian tubes and any enlargement of the ovaries. This information may help suggest the presence or absence of an infection.

The doctor may also take one or more blood samples to check for the presence of any antibodies to herpes or syphilis or for other organisms such as the AIDS virus (HIV), and hepatitis B and C.

What is involved in the physical examination (men)?

To enable an adequate examination, underpants should be removed and the foreskin rolled back (if you have not been circumcised). The doctor will then carefully examine the penis and testicles, checking for lumps, bumps, discharges, rashes and tenderness. He or she will also check for swelling of the lymph nodes in the groin and the epididymis.

Samples of any discharge will be collected for examination.

The doctor may also insert one or more small cotton buds into the eye of the penis to collect samples for testing.

An examination of the anus and throat may also be useful.

What if an STD is found?

If an STD is found, the doctor will suggest the appropriate treatment and discuss ways of reducing risk (such as altering your method of contraception and other ways of protecting yourself in the future). He or she will also suggest that, where possible, you contact any relevant sexual partner(s) to inform them of the need for an STD examination. You may wish to ask your doctor to make these approaches on your behalf.

For both men and women found to have an STD, a follow-up visit to the doctor is essential to determine whether any treatment given has been effective or if some other approach is necessary.

Until the doctor gives the 'all clear', you should avoid unprotected sexual intercourse as this may result in further STD spread.

A final important word

STDs are exactly that, **sexually transmitted**.

Thus any treatment must be given to **all** relevant partners.

If, after having been treated for an STD, you are exposed to the partner who infected you but who has not been treated, then re-infection is likely.

SUGGESTED FURTHER READING

Caplan P ed, *The cultural construction of sexuality*, Routledge, London, 1987.

Davenport-Hines R, *Sex, death and punishment*, Fontana Press, London, 1991

Bancroft J, *Human Sexuality and its problems*, Churchill Livingstone, Edinburgh, 1989

Gilbert GL ed, Infectious diseases: challenges for the 1900's. In: *Bailliere's Clinical Obstetrics and Gynaecology*, Vol 7, No 1, March 1993, Bailliere Tindall, London

Martin DH ed, Sexually Transmitted Diseases In: *The Medical Clinics of North America*, Vol 74, No 6, November 1990, W.B. Saunders, Philadelphia

Mindell A, Herpes simplex virus In: *Bloomsbury Series in Clinical Science*, Springer-verlag, London 1989

Mardh PA, The vaginal ecosystem, *American Journal of Obstetrics and Gynaecology* 1991, Vol 165, pp 1163-1168.

Plummer D, Garland S, Denham I, Chlamydia testing: a double blind exercise?, *Venereology* 1991, Vol 4, pp 63-64

Guillebaud J., *Contraception: your questions answered.* 2nd edition, 1990, Churchill Livingstone, Edinburgh

National Health and Medical Research Council, *Handbook on Sexually Transmitted Diseases*, 3rd edition, 1990, Commonweath of Australia, Canberra.

Centres for Disease Control, Sexually Transmitted Diseases Treatment Guidelines, *Morbidity and Mortality Weekly Report*, Vol 38 No S8 September 1989

Holmes KK, Mardh PA, Sparling PF et al eds, *Sexually Transmitted Diseases*, 2nd edition, 1990, McGraw-Hill Co, New York

Timewell E, Minichiello V, Plummer D., eds, *AIDS in Australia*, Prentice Hall, Sydney 1993

Bowden F ed, *The HIV Handbook*, Fairfield Hospital, Melbourne, 1992

INDEX

abdominal pain, 31, 32
abstinence, 21, 95
acetic acid test, 54
Acigel, 43
Acquired Immune Deficiency Syndrome
   see AIDS
acyclovir, 20, 61, 62, 66, 67
agar, 11
AIDS, 11, 15, 20, 89–103
   antibody test, 16
   Help Line, 96
   herpes and, 66
   opportunistic infections, 93, 99–102
   prevention, 94
   rashes and, 70
   tests, 94
   transmission during pregnancy, 110
allergies, 59
amoxicillin, 44
amphetamines, 80, 96
amphotericin, 101
ampicillin, 68
anaerobes, 43
anaphylaxis, 76
anorgasmia, 114
antibodies, 14, 15, 83
antibiotics, 11, 20, 21, 36–7, 74, 85,
   88-9, 107
antifungal treatments, 20
antigens, 14, 15, 39, 83
antiviral drugs, 20
anal intercourse, 30
anus, 2, 3
arthritis, 37, 109
AZT, 20, 97, 99

baby
   STD transmission to, 40, 110–11
bacteria, 9, 10, 11, 20
Bartholin's glands, 3, 52
B cell, 14
   lymphoma, 101
benzyl benzoate, 72
betadine antiseptic, 66

bilirubin, 78, 79
bimanual examination, 116
biopsy, 113
bladder, 6,7
   infections, 46–7
   problems, 45
blisters, 57, 60
blood supply
   testing for STDs, 92

Calymmatobacterium granulomatis, 67
cancer,
   AIDS-associated, 101, 102
   cervix, 3, 21, 32, 111–13
   rectum, 3
candida, 11, 20, 41-2, 72
carrier, 9, 13, 15, 80, 81
CD4 cells
   See helper T cells
CD8 cells
   See suppressor T cells
cefriaxone, 67
celibacy, 21
cerebral toxoplasmosis, 100
Cervical Intraepithelial Neoplasia (CIN),
   54, 111–13
cervicitis, 34, 35, 47
cervix, 3, 12
   cancer, 3, 21, 32, 49, 111–13
chancroid, 31, 57, 58, 67
Chlamydia trachomatis, 11, 12, 14, 15,
   16, 20, 22, 31, 32, 33, 34–40, 68, 106
   link with AIDS, 92
   transmission during childbirth, 111
ciprofloxacin, 37
circumcision, 6
cirrhosis, 21, 81
clitoris, 2
clotrimazole, 74, 75
'clue' cells, 43
codon, 10
cold sores, 63
   see also HPV
colposcopy, 54, 112

condoms, 21-2, 26, 27, 28, 29, 76, 95,
    108, 109
  animal gut, 60
  plastic, 60
  sensitivity to, 59
condylomata acuminata, 86
cone biopsy, 113
conjunctivitis, 109
corona, 6, 50
corticosteroids, 76, 82, 89
Corynebacterium minutissimum, 75
cotrimoxazole, 68, 97, 99, 100
crush preparation, 68
cryptococcus, 11, 20, 101
cryptosporidium, 12
culture
  of cells, 15, 38, 64
cyst, 51
cytomegalovirus (CMV), 79, 101

dapsone, 99, 100
'dark ground' microscopy, 16, 58, 85, 86
DDC, 97, 99
DDI, 97, 99
dendritic cells, 93
dental dams, 62
dermatitis, 58, 69, 75-7
dermatology, 69
dermatophytes, 12, 20
diabetes, 42, 74
diaphragm, 108, 109
diathermy, 55, 113
didanosine, 97,99
dideoxycytidine, 97, 99
discharge, 15, 16, 33-48
disinfectant, 59
DNA (Deoxyribo Nucleic Acid), 10
donavanosis, 57, 58, 67-8
double helix, 10
doxycycline, 20, 37, 40, 59, 68, 76, 89,
    90
drug use
  AIDS and, 95-7
dysplasia, 111
dysuria, 33

ectocervix, 3
ectopic pregnancy, 31, 32, 36, 105
eczema, 58
eggs (ova), 4
ejaculation, 6, 7
electron microscope, 16
ELISA, 39

endocarditis, 37
endocervix, 3
endometritis, 106
endometrium, 3
enzymes, 10
Epidermophyton, 73
epididymis, 7
epididymo-orchitis, 36, 37
Epstein Barr Virus (EBV), 79, 102
erection, 6, 8
erythrasma, 75
erythromycin, 20, 40, 67, 68, 75, 77, 89,
    111

Fallopian tubes, 4, 14, 31, 36
falloposcopy, 108
false negatives, 18, 19, 39
false positives, 18, 19, 39
fertility, 104-6
fever blisters, 63
fimbriae, 5
Fitz-Hugh-Curtis syndrome, 37
fixed drug reactions, 59, 76, 77
fluconazole, 42
foreskin, 6
frenulum, 6, 52, 53, 58
FTA test, 88, 90
fungus, 9, 10, 11, 20
  moulds, 11
  yeasts, 11

gamma benzene hexachloride, 72
gardnerella, 13, 16, 20, 41, 42-4, 46
generalised paresis of the insane (GPI),
    87
genetic code, 9, 10
glands
  swollen, 49-50
glandular fever, 11, 79
glans
  of penis, 6, 50
gonorrhoea, 11, 12, 15, 16, 20, 22, 23,
    24, 25, 31, 32, 34-41, 110-11
  in babies, 110-11
  symptoms, 35-7
  tests for, 38-9
  treatment, 37-8
gram stain, 16, 38, 41
granulomas, 68
griseofulvin, 74
gumma, 87

Haemophilus ducreyi, 67

hair follicles, 50--1
harm minimisation, 96-7
helper T cells, 14, 90, 97
hepatitis, 78-85
  carriers, 80, 81
  chronic, 80-1
  tests, 83-5
  vaccination, 80, 81
  type A, 79
  type B, 12, 15, 16, 21, 22, 79-85, 90,
    110
  type C, 11, 13, 21, 82, 84-5
  type D, 82-3, 85
  type E, 79
hepatoma, 81
heroin, 96
herpes, 11, 16, 20, 21, 22, 31, 32, 40, 41,
  44-5, 53, 57-67, 70, 76, 77
  chronic mucocutaneous tupe, 66
  diagnosis, 64-5
  link with AIDS, 92
  prevention, 65
  recurring, 61
  transmission during childbirth, 111
  treatment, 66-7
  type 1 (mouth herpes), 63
  type 2 (genital herpes), 63-4
  ulcers, 60
Herxheimer reaction, 89
heterosexuality
  STDs and, 31
HIV (Human Immunodeficiency Virus),
  11, 13, 14, 16, 20, 22, 31, 89-103
  antibody test, 94
  herpes and, 66
  testing for, 18-19
  transmission during pregnancy, 110
hives, 59, 76
homosexuality
  STDs and, 31
hormones, 4, 5, 8,
  oestrogen, 5,
  progesterone, 5,
  testosterone, 8
HPV (Human Papilloma Virus), 32, 49,
  52, 112
hymen, 2, 51
hysterectomy, 113

icterus, 78
IgG (Immunoglobulin G), 17
IgM (Immunoglobulin M), 17
immune deficiency

AIDS-associated, 89-90
immune
  dysfunction, 42
  system, 14
immunity, 14
immunofluorescence (IF), 39
immunoglobulin, 79, 81, 83
  M, 83
  G, 83
  total, 83
impotence, 114
incubation period, 60, 79
infections
  bladder, 46-7
  eye, 39
  kidney, 46
  rectum, 39
  throat, 39
infertility, 14, 21, 31, 32, 36, 37
inguinal nodes, 50
interferon, 82, 102
in vitro fertilisation (IVF), 37
irritants, 59, 70
IUD (intra uterine contraceptive device),
  31, 108
  risk of STDs and, 31

jaundice, 78, 80

Kaposi's sarcoma, 101
ketoconazole, 74
Koebner phenomenon, 70

labia majora, 2
labia minora, 2
lactobacilli, 43
laparoscopy, 107
laser treatment, 113, 55
lice, 12, 21, 69, 70-2
  eggs (nits), 71
liquid nitrogen,
  for warts, 55
liver
  damage, 21, 81
  function test, 85
lymphadenopathy, 86
lymph nodes
  enlarged, 49-50
  inguinal, 50
  painful, 68
  swollen, 68
lymphocyte, 14
Lymphogranuloma Venereum (LGV), 68

lymphoma, 101, 102

masturbation, 95
meatus, 40
meningitis, 61, 101
menopause, 4, 29
menstruation, 3
metronidazole, 20, 40, 44
micronazole, 74
Microsporum, 72
Mini Pill, 31, 108
Molluscum contageosum, 49, 56
monilia, 72
monogamy, 21–2, 95
mycobacteria, 100
myometrium, 3

needle exchange programs, 97
negative predictive value, 18
Neisseria gonorrhoea, 106
neurosyphilis, 87–8
nits, 71
non-specific urethritis (NSU), 38
    See also urethritis
nucleic acids, 9–10
nystatin, 42, 74

oestrogen, 5, 41, 52–3, 58
opportunistic infections, 93, 99, 102
oral sex, 30, 40
orchitis, 109
ova
    See eggs
ovaries, 4
overseas travel
    STDs and, 31–2
ovulation, 4, 5

pain
    abdominal, 31–2
    with urination, 33, 34–5
Pap smear, 3, 41, 49, 53, 54, 55,
    111–13, 115
parasites, 9, 10, 12, 21
para-urethral glands, 3
pearly penile papules, 50
Pediculus humanus, 70
pelvic inflammatory disease (PID), 32
    in men, 36, 106, 109
    in women, 36, 105–9
penicillin, 37, 88, 89, 111
    allergy to, 90
penis, 6, 12, 13

pentamidine, 100
peritonitis, 106
pessary, 20
photophobia, 61
photosensitivity, 76
PID
    See pelvic inflammatory disease
Pill, 31, 106, 108
pin worm, 12
pneumocystis pneumonia, 12, 100
pneumonia
    AIDS-associated, 98–9, 100
podophyllin, 55
polymorph, 38
positive predictive value, 18
pregnancy
    ectopic, 31, 32
prevention, 21–2, 94–7, 109
probenecid, 37
prodrome, 61, 79
progesterone, 5
prolapse, 29, 46
prostate, 6
    problems, 29, 36, 37, 109
prostitutes
    STDs and, 32
proteins, 10
    structural, 10
    enzymes, 10
protozoa, 12
psoriasis, 58, 69, 75
psychological impact
    of STDs, 1, 24–5, 26, 28–9, 51, 88,
        96, 98, 113–14
Pthirus pubis, 70
puberty, 4
pyosalpinx, 107
pyrimethamine, 100

reinfection, 20
ringworm, 73
RNA (Ribo Nucleic Acid), 10
Roman Catholic Church, 27
RPR (Rapid Plasma Reagin) test, 16, 88,
    89, 90

salpingitis, 106
sarcoptes scabei, 70
scabies, 1, 21, 69, 70–2
scrotum, 7
sebaceous glands, 50, 51–2
selenium sulphide, 75
semen, 6, 7

seminal vesibles, 7
sensitivity, 18
  to antibiotics, 37-8
septic arthritis, 37
seroconversion illness, 93
sex, 23-32, 40
  hormones, 5
smoking
  STDs and, 52
specificity, 18
'speed', 80, 96
sperm, 6
spermicide, 108, 109
spirochaete, 85
staphylococci, 13
STDs
  economic impact, 32
  historical aspects, 23-5
  risk assessment, 29-31
  transmission to babies, 110-11
sterility, 8
streptococci, 13
Stevens-Johnston syndrome, 59, 76
sulphonamides, 100
suppressor T cells, 14, 90, 97
syphilis, 11, 13, 15, 16, 20, 21, 24, 31, 32, 57, 69, 70, 85-89, 90
  chancre, 85-6
  gumma, 87
  latent, 87
  newborn, 89
  primary, 85
  secondary, 86
  tertiary, 87
  tests for, 86, 88
  transmission during pregnancy, 110, 111
  treatment, 88-9

tabes dorsalis, 87
T cells, 14
  T4 (CD4), 14, 90, 97
  T8 (CD8) 14, 90, 97
testicles, 7, 8
test tube baby program, 37
tetracyclines, 38, 59, 68, 76, 77, 111
thrush, 11, 13, 16, 20, 31, 41-2, 64, 69, 72, 74
  Pill use and, 31
tinea, 12, 20, 69, 72-5
  cruris, 73
  dermatophytes, 12, 20
  pedis, 73

versicolor, 75
tingling, 35, 61, 62, 77
tinidazole, 44
toxopasma, 12
toxoplasmosis, 100
TPHA test, 88
transformation zone, 3, 112
Treponaema pallidum, 85
trichomonas, 12, 16, 21, 40, 41, 44-5, 115
Trichophyton, 73
triplet, 10
tuberculosis (TB), 100, 101
Tyson's glands, 50

ulcers, 57, 60
  genital, 45
umbilication, 56
ureaplasmas, 40
urethra, 6, 7, 12
urethral meatus, 6
urethritis, 34, 40, 47, 109
urinary infections, 20
urine test, 16
uterus, 3

vaccines, 15
vagina, 2, 3, 13, 24
  discharge from, 103
  dry, 14, 24, 25, 29, 46, 60, 90
  examination of, 47, 115-16
  lubrication, 29
  oestrogen and, 41
  oestrogen creams for, 52-3
  prolapse, 45-6
  undiagnosed bleeding from, 99
vaginal intercourse, 30
vaginosis, 44
vas deferens, 7
venereology, 68
vesicles, 60
virus, 9, 10-11, 16, 20
vulva, 2, 13

wart, 49, 50, 51-6
  meatal, 40
  painting, 59
  structures resembling, 50-2, 86
  virus, 11, 12, 13-4, 21, 112
    See also HPV
'western blot' test, 18, 94
wet preparation, 16
window period, 17, 18

womb
  See uterus
wood's lamp, 75
wrestlers nodules, 56

xylocaine, 66

yeast, 11
  candida, 11, 13
  cryptococcus, 11
yoghurt, 43

zidovudine, 97, 99